User's Guide for the
SCID-5-PD
Structured Clinical Interview for
DSM-5® Personality Disorders

User's Guide for the

SCID-5-PD

Structured Clinical Interview for DSM-5® Personality Disorders

Also contains instructions for the
Structured Clinical Interview for DSM-5 Screening Personality Questionnaire

Michael B. First, M.D.
Professor of Clinical Psychiatry, Columbia University, and Research Psychiatrist,
Division of Clinical Phenomenology, New York State Psychiatric Institute,
New York, New York

Janet B.W. Williams, Ph.D.
Professor Emerita of Clinical Psychiatric Social Work (in Psychiatry and in
Neurology), Columbia University, and Research Scientist and Deputy Chief,
Biometrics Research Department (Retired), New York State Psychiatric Institute,
New York, New York; and Senior Vice President of Global Science,
MedAvante, Inc., Hamilton, New Jersey

Lorna Smith Benjamin, Ph.D.
Adjunct Professor of Psychiatry and Professor Emerita of Psychology,
University of Utah, Salt Lake City, Utah

Robert L. Spitzer, M.D.
Professor Emeritus of Psychiatry, Columbia University, and
Research Scientist and Chief, Biometrics Research Department (Retired),
New York State Psychiatric Institute, New York, New York

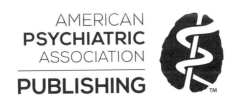

AMERICAN
PSYCHIATRIC
ASSOCIATION
PUBLISHING

If you wish to buy 50 or more copies of the same title, please go to www.appi.org/specialdiscounts for more information.

Manufactured in the United States of America on acid-free paper
23   6   5   4

Typeset in Palatino and Futura.

American Psychiatric Association Publishing
800 Maine Avenue SW, Suite 900
Washington, DC 20024-2812
www.appi.org

Contents

Acknowledgments vii

Citation and Additional Copyright Notices vii

Disclosures viii

1. Introduction 1

2. History 1

3. Features of the SCID-5-PD 2
   3.1 Coverage. 2
   3.2 Diagnostic Summary Score Sheet 2
   3.3 Basic Structure 3
   3.4 Screening Personality Questionnaire (SCID-5-SPQ). 5
   3.5 Deviations From DSM-5 Criteria 5

4. Administration of the SCID-5-PD. 6
   4.1 Sources of Information 6
   4.2 SCID-5-PD Interview Questions 6
   4.3 Interview Questions With Parenthetical Words in All-Capital Letters . . 7
   4.4 Ratings of Criterion Items 8
   4.5 Assessment of Other Specified Personality Disorder. 12
   4.6 Use of the SCID-5-PD With the SCID-5-SPQ 13
   4.7 Use of the SCID-5-PD Without the SCID-5-SPQ 15

5. SCID-5-PD Item-by-Item Commentary 15
   5.1 Avoidant Personality Disorder. 16
   5.2 Dependent Personality Disorder. 18
   5.3 Obsessive-Compulsive Personality Disorder 21
   5.4 Paranoid Personality Disorder. 24
   5.5 Schizotypal Personality Disorder 27
   5.6 Schizoid Personality Disorder. 31
   5.7 Histrionic Personality Disorder 34
   5.8 Narcissistic Personality Disorder 36
   5.9 Borderline Personality Disorder 39
   5.10 Antisocial Personality Disorder. 43

6. Training 48

7.   Reliability and Validity. 49
     7.1   Reliability of the SCID-5-PD 49
     7.2   Validity of the SCID-II. 51
     7.3   Psychometric Properties of the SCID-II Patient Questionnaire 52

References. 53

Appendix: SCID-5-SPQ and SCID-5-PD Example 55

Acknowledgments

We thank Rhonda Karg, our coauthor on the Structured Clinical Interview for DSM-5® Disorders—Research Version (SCID-5-RV) and the Structured Clinical Interview for DSM-5® Disorders—Clinician Version (SCID-5-CV) for her valuable contribution to the revision of the Structured Clinical Interview for DSM-5® Personality Disorders (SCID-5-PD) questions and her review of the *User's Guide for the Structured Clinical Interview for DSM-5 Personality Disorders.*

We also thank Desiree Caban, our research assistant and all-round jack-of-all-trades at Biometrics Research at Columbia University, for all of her invaluable assistance in helping to manage the development of the SCID-5-PD.

Finally, we would like to thank those at American Psychiatric Association Publishing who assisted in the production of the SCID-5-PD: Robert E. Hales, M.D., Editor-in-Chief; Rebecca Rinehart, Publisher; John McDuffie, Associate Publisher; Susan Westrate, Production Manager, for the careful typesetting of all elements and the cover and book design; and especially Ann. M. Eng, Senior Developmental Editor, whose meticulous and thoughtful editing helped ensure that the various details of this complex instrument fit together seamlessly.

Citation and Additional Copyright Notices

The Appendix case is adapted with permission from Spitzer RL, Gibbon M, Skodol AE, Williams JBW, First MB: *DSM-IV-TR Casebook: A Learning Companion to the Diagnostic and Statistical Manual of Mental Disorders, Fourth Edition, Text Revision*. Arlington, VA, American Psychiatric Publishing, 2002. Copyright © 2002. Used with permission.

Author's note: Some of the information describing the SCID-5-PD was adapted in part from: First MB, Spitzer RL, Gibbon M, Williams JBW: "The Structured Clinical Interview for DSM-III-R Personality Disorders (SCID-II), Part I: Description." *Journal of Personality Disorders* 9:2, June 1995.

Disclosures

The following authors have declared all forms of support received within the 12 months prior to manuscript submittal that may represent a competing interest in relation to their work published in this volume, as follows:

Lorna Smith Benjamin, Ph.D., is the author of Structural Analysis of Social Behavior (SASB) models, questionnaires, and software, which are owned by University of Utah. She is the author of *Interpersonal Diagnosis and Treatment of Personality Disorders*, New York, Guilford Press, 1993, 1996, 2003; and author of *Interpersonal Reconstructive Therapy*, New York, Guilford Press, 2003, 2006.

Janet B. W. Williams, Ph.D., works full-time as the Senior Vice President of Global Science, MedAvante, Inc., a pharmaceuticals services company.

The following authors of this work have no competing interests to report:

Michael B. First, M.D.; Robert L. Spitzer, M.D.

1. Introduction

The Structured Clinical Interview for DSM-5 Personality Disorders (SCID-5-PD) is a semistructured diagnostic interview for assessing the 10 DSM-5 Personality Disorders in Clusters A, B, and C. The SCID-5-PD was formerly called the Structured Clinical Interview for DSM-IV Axis II Personality Disorders (SCID-II; see the "History" section below for more information). The SCID-5-PD can be used to make Personality Disorder diagnoses, either categorically (present or absent) or dimensionally (summing the ratings [0, 1, or 2] for each diagnosis and treating these sums as dimensions).

The SCID-5-PD can also be used in several different types of studies, as was the SCID-II. Some studies have used it to investigate patterns of Personality Disorders co-occurring with other mental disorders (e.g., Casadio et al. 2014; Mulder et al. 2010; Odlaug et al. 2012; Williams et al. 2010) or medical conditions (e.g., Calderone et al. 2015; Uguz et al. 2008). Other studies (Edens et al. 2015; Gremaud-Heitz et al. 2014; Martín-Blanco et al. 2014) have used it to select a group of study subjects with a particular Personality Disorder (e.g., Antisocial Personality Disorder, Borderline Personality Disorder). Finally, other studies have used it to investigate the underlying structure of personality pathology (e.g., Sharp et al. 2015) and for comparison with other assessment methods for personality disorders (e.g., Huprich et al. 2015; Rojas et al. 2014).

2. History

The origins of the SCID-5-PD can be traced back to the early developmental stages of the Structured Clinical Interview for DSM-III (SCID) that included a personality disorders module developed by Jeffrey Jonas, M.D., of McLean Hospital in the 1984 version of the SCID. In 1985, this personality disorders module was reformulated into a separate, stand-alone instrument (called the SCID-II) because of the length of the module, burgeoning research interest in personality disorders, and the special assessment requirements for personality features. In 1986, the SCID-II was updated for DSM-III-R and a new strategy, with a screening personality questionnaire (the SCID-II-PQ), was incorporated. After field trials establishing the reliability of the SCID-II were completed (First et al. 1995), a final version of the SCID-II for DSM-III-R Personality Disorders (Spitzer et al. 1990) was published by American Psychiatric Press as a component of the SCID. After the publication of DSM-IV (American Psychiatric Association 1994), work was begun on revising the SCID-II. With the help of Lorna Benjamin, Ph.D., many of the SCID-II questions were reworded to make them more reflective of the subject's inner experience. The DSM-IV version of the SCID-II (First et al. 1997) was published by American Psychiatric Press.

After the publication of DSM-5 in 2013, work began on revising the SCID-II, which has been rechristened the SCID-5-PD to reflect the fact that Personality Disorders are no longer listed on Axis II given the elimination of the multiaxial system in DSM-5. Although none of the DSM-IV Personality Disorder criteria were changed in DSM-5, all of the SCID-5-PD interview questions were reviewed with an eye toward ensuring that the wording of the questions was optimal for capturing the construct embodied in the diagnostic criteria, resulting in a number of wording changes. Moreover, the assessments of the DSM-IV research categories Passive-Aggressive Personality Disorder (Negativistic Personality Disorder) and Depressive Personality Disorder were removed from the SCID-5-PD, given their elimination as research categories in DSM-5.

3. Features of the SCID-5-PD

3.1 Coverage

The SCID-5-PD covers all 10 of the DSM-5 Personality Disorders (in Clusters A, B, and C), as well as Other Specified Personality Disorder. Ordinarily the entire SCID-5-PD is administered; however, it is also possible to evaluate only those Personality Disorders that are of particular interest to the clinician or researcher.

3.2 Diagnostic Summary Score Sheet

The SCID-5-PD Diagnostic Summary Score Sheet is located at the very beginning of the SCID-5-PD for ease of use. It is not until the conclusion of the SCID-5-PD that the interviewer completes the Diagnostic Summary Score Sheet, which summarizes the results of the evaluation of each of the 10 DSM-5 Personality Disorders plus Other Specified Personality Disorder. For each Personality Disorder, the interviewer first indicates whether the categorical threshold has been met (e.g., at least 4 out of 7 criteria for Avoidant Personality Disorder) under the column labeled "Categorical criteria met?" If the categorical threshold has not been met for a particular disorder, the interviewer can still indicate the presence of clinically significant subthreshold features of that disorder under the column labeled "If criteria not met, are there clinically significant features?"

The SCID-5-PD also includes a provision for making a dimensional rating for each of the DSM-5 Personality Disorder categories by summing up the individual scores for the ratings and circling the appropriate number. Although this is not an official feature of the DSM-5 Personality Disorder classification, the idea of dimensionalizing the categorical disorders in this way has been proposed by researchers (e.g., Oldham and Skodol 2000) as a potentially useful addition to the categorical classification. For each disorder, the interviewer sums up all of the ratings ("0," "1," and "2"), producing a dimensional score for that disorder that reflects both threshold and subthreshold ratings for the criteria. Note that the highest possible dimensional score for each Personality Disorder is twice the total number of possible criteria, because scores of "0," "1," and "2" are being summed across the Personality Disorder items. Because the total number of criteria vary from disorder to disorder, the spacing between the score points also varies so that the equivalent levels of severity line up across the dimensional representations of the disorders.

In the common situation in which the criteria for more than one Personality Disorder are met, the rater is instructed to indicate the "principal Personality Disorder diagnosis" (i.e., the Personality Disorder that is, or should be, the main focus of clinical attention) by recording the ICD-10-CM code (located to the left of each diagnosis on the score sheet) on the bottom of the score sheet.

3.3 Basic Structure

The basic structure of the SCID-5-PD is similar to that of the other SCID-5 interviews that cover non–personality disorders (e.g., the SCID-5 Research Version [SCID-5-RV]; the SCID-5 Clinician Version [SCID-5-CV]). Modeled on the clinical interview, the SCID-5-PD begins with an overview that records background information about the subject that is useful in making the ratings of the individual Personality Disorder criteria. The SCID-5-PD overview has two sections:

- The first section, labeled "General Overview," starts with the collection of basic demographic data (e.g., age, marital status, living situation), education and work history, history of interactions with the legal system, and then finally a brief summary of current and past periods of psychopathology. The SCID-5-PD is often administered following a SCID-5-RV or SCID-5-CV evaluation, which may have been given on a previous occasion. When the SCID-5-PD is administered after the SCID-5-RV (or SCID-5-CV), the General Overview can be skipped because it covers the same information as the overview sections in the SCID-5-RV or SCID-5-CV, albeit in more detail. Either way, it is important for the interviewer to determine whether there have been any circumscribed periods during which another psychiatric disorder, such as an episode of Major Depressive Disorder, may have occurred.
- The second section of the overview, labeled "Overview for Assessment of Personality Disorders," aims to characterize the subject's usual behavior and relationships and also provides information about the subject's capacity for self-reflection. It starts with the statement: "Now I am going to ask you some questions about the kind of person you are—that is, how you generally have felt or behaved." This is followed by a number of open-ended questions intended to assess general personality characteristics (e.g., "How would you describe yourself as a person? How successful would you say you are at getting the things you want in life, like having a satisfying relationship, a fulfilling career, or close friends? If you could change your personality in some way, how would you want to be different?"). If there have been any current or past periods of psychopathology (as determined by completion of a SCID interview for non–personality disorders or as determined during the General Overview), the interviewer instructs the subject to consider those times when the psychiatric disorder has *not* been present when answering the SCID-5-PD questions.

After the overview sections, the interview proceeds with questions assessing the DSM-5 criteria for each of the 10 specific Personality Disorders, in turn: Avoidant Personality Disorder, Dependent Personality Disorder, Obsessive-Compulsive Personality Disorder, Paranoid Personality Disorder, Schizotypal Personality Disorder, Schizoid Personality Disorder, Histrionic Personality Disorder, Narcissistic Personality Disorder, Borderline Personality Disorder, and Antisocial Personality Disorder. The order of the

Personality Disorders in the SCID-5-PD differs from that in DSM-5 to enhance rapport with the subject. Thus, the SCID-5-PD does not begin with questions for the Cluster A "odd or eccentric" features grouping (i.e., Paranoid, Schizoid, and Schizotypal Personality Disorders), but rather with the Cluster C "anxious or fearful" grouping (i.e., Avoidant, Dependent, and Obsessive-Compulsive Personality Disorders). Moreover, the assessment of Antisocial Personality Disorder (in the Cluster B "dramatic, emotional, or erratic" grouping) is left for last given its potential negative impact on rapport. Finally, the SCID-5-PD concludes with the opportunity for the interviewer to make a diagnosis of Other Specified Personality Disorder for cases in which personality disorder features from several Personality Disorders are present that do not meet the full criteria for any specific disorder, yet cause significant impairment in functioning.

Mirroring the interview layout of the SCID-5-RV and SCID-5-CV, the SCID-5-PD assessment of each of the DSM-5 Personality Disorders has three columns. The left-hand column of each page of the SCID-5-PD consists of the SCID-5-PD interview questions (in bold) and directions (in all-capital letters) for the interviewer. The DSM-5 diagnostic criteria to which the interview questions refer are in the gray-shaded middle column of the page. The right-hand column of each page contains the codes for rating the criteria: "?"=Inadequate information, "0"=Absent, "1"=Subthreshold, and "2"=Threshold. (See Section 4.4, "Ratings of Criterion Items," for a discussion of the factors that should be considered in making a rating of "2.") It should be emphasized that (as with the SCID-5-RV and SCID-5-CV) the ratings reflect the interviewer's judgment regarding whether or not the DSM-5 diagnostic criterion in the center column is met, not just the subject's answer to the interview questions for that criterion. Frequently the subject will answer "YES" to an interview question, but the interviewer's clinical judgment (after further inquiry) will be that the criterion should be rated "0" or "1."

In the gray-shaded middle column of the SCID-5-PD, the DSM-5 diagnostic criteria occasionally contain a "(**Note**)" in parentheses; this reflects the inclusion of such notes as they are contained in the DSM-5 criteria. Other notes, italicized and enclosed in brackets, have been added to the SCID-5-PD to reduce the potential for false-positive ratings. For example, below Criterion 5 in Dependent Personality Disorder (i.e., "Goes to excessive lengths to obtain nurturance and support from others, to the point of volunteering to do things that are unpleasant"), a *"[Note]"* advises the interviewer "Do not include behavior intended to achieve goals other than being liked, such as job advancement."

The far right-hand column of the SCID-5-PD includes consecutively numbered field codes, one for each rated entity in the SCID-5-PD. Although the primary purpose of the field codes is to provide a standardized way of referring to SCID-5-PD data items to facilitate comparison of SCID-5-PD results from different studies, these field codes are also useful in SCID-5-PD supervision for referring to individual, rated items during discussion of the ratings.

3.4   Screening Personality Questionnaire (SCID-5-SPQ)

A feature of the SCID-5-PD is the availability of a self-report personality questionnaire as a screening tool to shorten the time that it takes the clinician to administer the instrument. Subjects usually need about 20 minutes to complete the Structured Clinical Interview for DSM-5 Screening Personality Questionnaire (SCID-5-SPQ). Afterward, the SCID-5-PD interview is administered, with the clinician needing to inquire only about the items screened positive ("YES" answers) on the SCID-5-SPQ. The assumption is that a subject who responds with a "NO" on the SCID-5-SPQ item would also have answered "NO" to the same SCID-5-PD question had it been asked aloud by the interviewer.

The SCID-5-SPQ requires an eighth-grade or higher reading level (as determined by the Flesch-Kincaid formula). Each of the 106 questions in the SCID-5-SPQ corresponds to an initial interview question in the SCID-5-PD (identified by numbers in the left-hand column of both instruments). For example, Question 78 in the SCID-5-SPQ is, "Do relationships with people you really care about have lots of extreme ups and downs?" This corresponds to the initial SCID-5-PD interview Question 78 for the second criterion in Borderline Personality Disorder. In most cases, the items in the SCID-5-SPQ set a threshold for a positive response that is considerably lower than that of the corresponding diagnostic criterion in the SCID-5-PD. For example, Question 52 in the SCID-5-SPQ asks, "Do you like being the center of attention?" It is expected that a number of individuals will circle "YES" on the SCID-5-SPQ although, on further questioning during the SCID-5-PD interview, the corresponding criterion, "Is uncomfortable in situations in which he or she is not the center of attention," will not be met. In other words, the SCID-5-SPQ acts as a low-threshold screening device with intentionally high rates of false positives. It is also expected that there will be few false negatives resulting from the SCID-5-SPQ, because the interviewer is encouraged to explore items for which any evidence emerges during the SCID-5-PD interview, regardless of the subject's response on the SCID-5-SPQ (e.g., asking about suspiciousness if the subject acts suspicious during the interview even though the subject may have denied it on the SCID-5-SPQ). Because of the intended high false-positive rates, we do not recommend using the SCID-5-SPQ as a stand-alone instrument for any purpose other than as a rough screening device.

3.5   Deviations From DSM-5 Criteria

For editorial reasons, we retained the DSM-IV convention of capitalizing disorder names so as to more clearly set off these diagnostic constructs from the rest of the text. For similar reasons, we also decided to retain the DSM-IV term "general medical condition" (GMC) throughout the SCID-5 instructions to refer to medical conditions listed outside the mental disorders chapter in the International Classification of Diseases (ICD), rather than use the DSM-5 term "another medical condition." However, we retained the use of "another medical condition" when it appears within a DSM-5 diagnostic criterion.

4. Administration of the SCID-5-PD

4.1   Sources of Information

Most typically, the subject of the SCID-5-PD interview is the sole source of information; however, the interviewer should use any sources available when making the ratings, including information from a current or previous therapist and from family members or other informants. Ancillary information may be especially important in the evaluation of Personality Disorders because of a tendency for subjects to underreport personality pathology. Although not specifically designed for this purpose, the SCID-5-PD can be administered to an informant (e.g., therapist, family member, close friend) about the subject. In cases in which contradictory information is elicited, the interviewer must use his or her clinical judgment in determining whether the informant or the subject is giving the more valid account.

4.2   SCID-5-PD Interview Questions

Any number preceding a SCID-5-PD interview question indicates that the same-numbered question is also included in the self-report SCID-5-SPQ. (See Section 3.4 for a discussion of how to use the SCID-5-PD with the SCID-5-SPQ.) Because the purpose of the SCID-5-SPQ is to allow the interviewer to bypass the evaluation of a Personality Disorder criterion during the SCID-5-PD interview if the question has been answered "NO" on the SCID-5-SPQ—and there is no indication from the subject's behavior during the interview to suggest that the item might be present—the SCID-5-SPQ questions have been written rather broadly to encourage overrreporting in order to maximize their sensitivity and minimize the risk of false negatives. Thus, additional follow-up questions in the SCID-5-PD (which usually involve asking the subject to provide additional clarifying information or illustrative examples) are necessary to determine whether the Personality Disorder criterion is actually met at a threshold level of severity. For example, the first question in the SCID-5-PD interview (numbered 1 in the left-hand column of the SCID-5-PD and the SCID-5-SPQ), asks whether the subject has avoided jobs or tasks that involved having to deal with a lot of people. Because the actual DSM-5 criterion requires that the person avoid occupational activities that involve significant interpersonal contact because of fears of criticism, disapproval, or rejection, it is necessary to ask follow-up questions in order to determine first whether the jobs or tasks that are avoided do involve significant interpersonal contact (i.e., "Give me some examples"), and then to determine the reason why the person avoids those activities—i.e., "What was the reason that you avoided these (JOBS OR TASKS)? (Is it because you just don't like to be around people, or is it because you are afraid of being criticized or rejected?").

Most of the Personality Disorder criteria have only one left-numbered SCID-5-PD interview question that corresponds to each criterion. Some of the criteria, however, particularly those that may be more difficult to assess in an interview format (e.g., identity disturbance in Borderline Personality Disorder, field code PD77), have several left-numbered SCID-5-PD interview questions (e.g., Questions 79–82) that attempt to address different aspects of the criterion. In such cases, the interviewer should ask as many of these left-numbered questions as needed in order to gather enough information to determine whether the criterion should be rated a "2." For example, three numbered questions (Questions 33–35) are provided for the assessment of the first criterion for Schizotypal Personality Disorder (i.e., "ideas of reference," field code PD36). If the subject provides enough convincing examples of referential thinking in response to the first question (i.e., Question 33, "When you are out in public and see people talking, do you often feel that they are talking about you?"), there is no need to ask the other two questions (Questions 34 and 35) as well. However, if the answer to Question 33 is negative (or the examples are deemed by the interviewer to be insufficient to justify a threshold rating of "2"), Questions 34 and 35 must be asked in addition to Question 33.

SCID-5-PD questions not enclosed in parentheses are to be asked verbatim of every subject. Questions in parentheses should be asked when necessary to clarify responses and can be skipped if the interviewer already either knows the answer to the parenthetical question or has sufficient information to rate the criterion as "2." For example, in the assessment of Obsessive-Compulsive Personality Disorder, Criterion 7 ("Adopts a miserly spending style toward both self and others; money is viewed as something to be hoarded for future catastrophes"), following the initial question (Question 22, field code PD24) asking the subject if it is hard for him to spend money on himself and other people, the interviewer is instructed to ask the subject "Why?" The parenthetical questions following this ("Is this because you're worried about not having enough in the future when you might really need it? What might you need it for?") only need to be asked if the subject's explanation for why he finds it difficult to spend money suggests a different motivation than wanting to hoard money as a hedge against a future catastrophe. The fact that a question is in parentheses does not imply that the information the question is designed to elicit is any less critical. In most cases, the parenthetical questions reflect information that is likely to have already been elicited by earlier questions.

For most items, the interviewer should ask the subject to provide specific details of thoughts, feelings, and behaviors to support the criterion ratings. This information should be recorded in the SCID-5-PD in order to document the information used to justify the interviewer's rating. The interviewer should clearly label information that was obtained from sources other than the subject (e.g. charts, specific informant).

4.3   Interview Questions With Parenthetical Words in All-Capital Letters

Some of the SCID-5-PD questions contain phrases in all-capital letters enclosed in parentheses—e.g., "(JOBS OR TASKS)," (SXS OF PSYCHOTIC DISORDER)," "(ANTISOCIAL ACTS)," "(INCLUDING SPOUSE OR PARTNER)." This convention indicates that the interviewer is to modify the question and insert the specific information provided by the subject or informants in place of these capital-letter designations, usually in the person's own words. For example, in Antisocial Personality Disorder, the first question in the assessment of Criterion A7 (i.e., lack of remorse; field code PD108) is

"How do you feel about (ANTISOCIAL ACTS)?" In this case, the interviewer substitutes the actual antisocial acts that the subject has admitted to doing in the context of the evaluation of the prior six Criterion A items for Antisocial Personality Disorder (e.g., "How do you feel about having stolen money from your brother, forging his checks, and totaling his car while you were high on cocaine?").

4.4   Ratings of Criterion Items

The DSM-5 Personality Disorder criteria require that the pattern of inner experience or behavior has been present at a sufficient level of severity, persistence, and pervasiveness in order to count toward the diagnosis. For the individual Personality Disorder criteria, the SCID-5-PD offers four possible ratings: "?"=Inadequate information, "0"=Absent, "1"=Subthreshold, and "2"=Threshold.

?=Inadequate information to rate the criterion as either "0," "1," or "2"
A rating of "?" should be reserved for those relatively rare situations in which there is insufficient information for a more definitive rating for the criterion, such as when the subject answers "YES" to a SCID-5-PD question but is unable to recall any illustrative examples. For example, in the evaluation of Criterion 1 for Narcissistic Personality Disorder ("Has a grandiose sense of self-importance"; field code PD65), a subject answers "YES" to Question 61 ("Have people told you that you have too high an opinion of yourself?") but then says that he cannot recall any actual examples when this has happened. A rating of "?" may also be given temporarily to indicate uncertainty about the rating pending additional information from informants.

0=Absent
A rating of "0" is made when the pattern of inner experience or behavior described in the criterion is clearly absent.

1=Subthreshold
A rating of "1" is made when the pattern of inner experience or behavior covered in the criterion is present but below the diagnostic threshold in terms of severity, persistence, or pervasiveness. (See guidelines for a rating of "2," below.) For example, in the evaluation of Criterion 1 for Borderline Personality Disorder ("Frantic efforts to avoid real or imagined abandonment"; field code PD75), a rating of "1" would be appropriate for a subject who answered "YES" to SCID-5-PD Question 77 ("Have you become frantic when you thought that someone you really cared about was going to leave you?") and described pleading with an ex-boyfriend not to leave and then reported that it happened only in some of her past relationships, but not others.

2=Threshold
A rating of "2" is made when the pattern of inner experience or behavior described in the criterion is present at a threshold or pathological level of severity. To facilitate the differentiation of a rating of subthreshold ("1") from a rating of threshold ("2"),

below each criterion in the center column of the SCID-5-PD is a specific guideline for making a "2" rating. Moreover, in addition to the criterion-specific guidelines for "2" ratings, each of the following criteria for general personality disorder (DSM-5 pp. 646–647; summarized in the SCID-5-PD section "General Personality Disorder Criteria That Should Be Considered When Making a Rating of "2," pages 5–6) should be considered when determining whether a particular Personality Disorder criterion warrants a rating of "2," as described additionally here.

General Personality Disorder Criteria That Should Be Considered When Making a Rating of "2"

A. An enduring pattern of inner experience and behavior that deviates markedly from the expectations of the individual's culture. All personality traits occur on a continuum. This general criterion highlights the fact that by definition, a Personality Disorder criterion must be at the extreme end of that continuum for it to warrant a rating of "2." For example, some degree of social anxiety with unfamiliar people is present in most people; however, Criterion 9 (field code PD44) of Schizotypal Personality Disorder ("excessive social anxiety that does not diminish with familiarity and tends to be associated with paranoid fears rather than negative judgments about self") would be rated "2" only if the subject acknowledges that the anxiety continues even after knowing other people for a while and that the anxiety is related to suspiciousness about other peoples' motives. Moreover, this general criterion also underscores the fact that an individual's impairment in personality functioning may be at least partly due to a clash between the expression of an individual's personality and the expectations of his or her cultural milieu. These follow-up questions may be helpful in determining whether the subject's pattern of inner experience and behavior deviates markedly from cultural norms:

> What is that like?
> Give me some examples.
> Do you think you are more this way than most people you know?

B. The enduring pattern is inflexible and pervasive across a broad range of personal and social situations. In order to justify a rating of "2," there must be evidence that the enduring pattern of behavior, cognition, or affect is both inflexible and pervasive. The inflexible nature of a personality trait results in the expression of the pattern consistently across most situations. Therefore, the interviewer should look for evidence that the trait has a pervasive impact on all (or most) areas of personality functioning and is not restricted to a single interpersonal relationship, situation, or role. If the pattern of behavior, cognition, or affect has occurred only in the context of interacting with one person but not with most others (e.g., with a particular boss but not with all supervisors, with one ex-boyfriend but not most others), it is more likely to represent a relational problem or an Adjustment Disorder than a personality trait. These follow-up questions may be helpful:

Does this happen in a lot of different situations?
Does this happen with a lot of different people?

C.   The enduring pattern leads to clinically significant distress or impairment in social, occupational, or other important areas of functioning.   The impairment in personality functioning resulting from the enduring pattern of inner experience and behavior occurs on a continuum. Only when a personality trait is maladaptive and thus causes significant functional impairment or subjective distress, does it warrant a rating of "2." The interviewer should ask questions to determine the negative impact of the trait on the subject's social interactions, his ability to form and maintain close relationships, and his ability to function effectively at work, school, or home. These follow-up questions may be helpful:

What problems has this caused for you?
Has this affected your relationships or your interactions with other people?
   (How about your family, romantic partner, or friends?)
Has this affected your work/school?
Has it bothered other people?

Because personality traits are commonly ego-syntonic (i.e., they involve characteristics that the person experiences as an integral part of the self) or have been so long-standing that their negative impact on functioning is no longer apparent, the subject may deny that the trait has any negative impact on his functioning. For example, individuals with Obsessive-Compulsive Personality Disorder may find their perfectionism and incessant devotion to work to be a cherished quality and an indication of scrupulousness, moral superiority, and dedication. It is important to recognize that subjective distress or a direct acknowledgment of impairment is *not* necessary for a rating of "2." If, in the interviewer's clinical opinion, the trait is having a significantly negative impact on the subject's level of functioning, the criterion should be rated "2." For example, if a person with no friends who has not been able to advance in his career because of social avoidance rationalizes that he prefers being alone and working in a low-level job, this would warrant a "2" rating of Criterion 1 (field code PD1) for Avoidant Personality Disorder ("Avoids occupational activities that involve significant interpersonal contact").

D.   The pattern is stable and of long duration, and its onset can be traced back at least to adolescence or early adulthood.   Personality traits do not refer to time-limited and discrete episodes of illness. Rather, maladaptive personality traits are by definition chronic patterns with an early and insidious onset evident by late adolescence or early adulthood. For the purposes of the SCID-5-PD, the concept of "long duration" is operationalized so that a rating of "2" means that the characteristic has been frequently present over a period of at least the last 5 years. (The only exceptions are certain extreme items, such as suicidal behavior, that are diagnostically significant even when they occur relatively infrequently.) Furthermore, there must be some evidence of the trait going back as far as the subject's late teens or early 20s. These follow-up questions may be helpful:

> Have you been this way for a long time?
> How often does this happen?
> When can you first remember (feeling/acting) this way? (Do you remember a
>   period of time when you didn't feel this way?)

E. The enduring pattern is not better explained as a manifestation or consequence of another mental disorder.   The evaluation of Personality Disorders in the presence of other psychiatric conditions is often quite difficult. A subject's current behavior may result more from the presence of an episodic Mood or Anxiety Disorder than from a stable personality disposition. In order to tease out the relationships between Personality Disorders and other psychiatric conditions, the interviewer must confirm that the trait has been present and long-standing prior to and independent of any other psychiatric conditions.

When determining whether a criterion should be rated "2" in the presence of another mental disorder with symptoms that resemble the personality trait in question, it may be helpful to ask the following question: Are you generally this way even when you are not (SYMPTOM OF OTHER DISORDER, e.g., depressed)? In cases in which the non–personality disorder itself has been long-standing and persistent, trying to determine whether the behavior is part of the disorder or better considered to be a personality trait may be impossible (and ultimately meaningless). In such situations, it probably makes the most sense NOT to attribute the trait to the other mental disorder and to make a rating of "2."

F. The enduring pattern is not attributable to the physiological effects of a substance (e.g., a drug of abuse, a medication) or another medical condition (e.g., head trauma).   The relationship between some Personality Disorders (particularly Borderline and Antisocial Personality Disorders) and substance use can be difficult to evaluate. In some people, substance use may be indicative of the impulsivity that is characteristic of these Personality Disorders or may be a form of self-medication to regulate the dysphoric mood states that may be associated with them. In other people, the behaviors that seem to characterize the "personality disorder" may in fact be secondary to drug taking, either by direct physiological effect (e.g., the substance causes affective lability) or the fact that obtaining the funds for illegal substances often entails antisocial behavior. In such situations, a careful evaluation comparing the onset of the personality traits and the pattern of substance use may be helpful in teasing out their relationship. The following questions may be helpful in determining the relationship between the substance use and personality functioning in individuals who have a history of prolonged excessive alcohol or drug use:

> Does this happen only when you are drunk or high or withdrawing from alcohol or
> drugs? Does this happen only when you are trying to get alcohol or drugs?

The other part of this criterion refers to the differential diagnosis between a Personality Disorder and Personality Change Due to Another Medical Condition. Although a number of GMCs can result in personality changes, in practice this differential diagnosis is rarely a problem because of the difference in characteristic age and mode of onset between a Personality Disorder and Personality Change Due to Another Medical Condition. In Personality Disorders, there must be an early and usually gradual onset that is not related to a GMC. In Personality Change Due to Another Medical Condition, the onset can be at any age and must be a direct result of the effects of a GMC on the central nervous system. The situation in which this differential may be most difficult is when the "personality change" occurs in childhood and is not conclusively related to the GMC. For example, it may be difficult to evaluate whether symptoms of Conduct Disorder occurring in a child who had preexisting head trauma are due to the head injury or whether the injury is incidental.

One final caveat.   It is important to keep in mind that interviewers have their own enduring styles of personality functioning that may color their perceptions and judgments of the personality functioning of others. For example, an interviewer with obsessive-compulsive traits may have difficulty appreciating the pathological nature of such traits when these are present in others, but may be excessively judgmental in evaluating subjects with histrionic features. Social, cultural, and gender biases can further complicate the assessment. For example, interviewers from cultures that place a high value on controlled and compulsive behavior are more likely to see as pathologically histrionic the more spontaneous behavior sanctioned by other cultures, and vice versa. Furthermore, interviewers (whether male or female) may at times be influenced by their stereotypes about "normal" masculine and feminine behavior. It is therefore important that the interviewer be aware of the possible effects of his or her own biases when determining whether a particular behavior, cognition, or affect is "pathological" and deserving of a rating of "2."

In summary: remember the three Ps.   The fundamental requirements for deciding whether behavior, cognition, or affect should be considered evidence of a Personality Disorder and thus warrant a rating of "2" can be summarized as follows. A rating of "2" requires that the behavior, cognition, or affect be

- **Pathological** (i.e., outside the range of normal variation)
- **Persistent** (i.e., frequently present over a period of at least the last 5 years with onset by early adulthood)
- **Pervasive** (i.e., apparent in a variety of contexts, such as at work and at home, or in the case of items concerning interpersonal relations, occurring in several different relationships)

4.5   Assessment of Other Specified Personality Disorder

At the conclusion of the assessment of Antisocial Personality Disorder, the interviewer needs to consider whether a diagnosis of Other Specified Personality Disorder is appropriate. In DSM-5 (p. 684), Other Specified Personality Disorder is defined as "presentations in which symptoms characteristic of a Personality Disorder…predominate but do not meet the full criteria for any of the disorders in the Personality Disorders diagnostic class." Most commonly, this category is used when there are features characteristic of specific DSM-5 Personality Disorders but not enough to reach the diagnostic threshold for any one of them. For example, when the features are characteristic of only one of the specific Personality Disorders (e.g., Narcissistic Personality Disorder), then Other Specified Personality Disorder is diagnosed to indicate a subthreshold version of that disorder that is still sufficiently severe to cause clinically significant impairment in functioning. Or more commonly, features from several different specific Personality Disorders are present (i.e., "mixed personality features"), each at a subthreshold level. In either of these cases, the presence of subthreshold features is indicated on the SCID-5-PD Diagnostic Summary Score Sheet in the column "If criteria not met, are there clinically significant features?" (to the right of the column "Categorical criteria for a disorder met?"). Finally, Other Specified Personality Disorder may also be appropriate for personality disturbances that do not conform to any of the DSM-5 Personality Disorders (e.g., Passive-Aggressive Personality Disorder from DSM-IV Appendix B "Criteria Sets and Axes Provided for Further Study"). In such cases, the name of the non-DSM-5 personality disorder is recorded in the "Other Specified Personality Disorder" row of the SCID-5-PD Diagnostic Summary Score Sheet.

4.6   Use of the SCID-5-PD With the SCID-5-SPQ

The SCID-5-SPQ may be given to the subject to fill out before the interviewer administers the SCID-5-PD (see also Section 3.4, "Screening Personality Questionnaire (SCID-5-SPQ)," and Section 4.2, "SCID-5-PD Interview Questions," in this User's Guide). It is sometimes helpful to send the SCID-5-SPQ to the subject by mail before the scheduled SCID-5-PD interview, asking the subject to bring in the completed questionnaire to the SCID-5-PD interview session. Before commencing the SCID-5-PD interview, the interviewer reviews the completed SCID-5-SPQ, circling the left-numbered questions on the SCID-5-PD that correspond to the same left-numbered questions circled "YES" on the SCID-5-SPQ. If a SCID-5-SPQ question is not answered at all (i.e., neither "YES" nor "NO" is circled), then the question number should be circled in the SCID-5-PD *and* a question mark added in writing to the left of the SCID-5-PD question number. Once all "YES" and unanswered questions are noted on the left-hand side of the SCID-5-PD, the interviewer proceeds with the SCID-5-PD as follows:

1. For all questions preceded by a circled number (i.e., indicating that the question was answered "YES" on the SCID-5-SPQ), the interviewer asks the SCID-5-PD question, leaving out the italicized text in brackets. The SCID-5-PD question is a paraphrased version of the screening question (i.e., "You've said that…"), acknowledging that the subject answered the corresponding SCID-5-SPQ question "YES."
2. For all questions preceded by an uncircled number (i.e. indicating a "NO" answer on the SCID-5-SPQ), the question is *not* asked and the corresponding criterion is

rated "0." (Note: the interviewer should rate a "0" only if confident that this is a true negative—see discussion later in this section for two exceptions).

3. For all questions preceded by a circled number accompanied by a question mark (i.e., indicating that the question was neither answered "YES" nor "NO" on the SCID-5-SPQ), the interviewer asks the SCID-5-PD question, starting with the italicized text in brackets that corresponds to the wording of the original SCID-5-SPQ question.

To illustrate the application of these options, the left-numbered SCID-5-PD Question 1 (which corresponds to Criterion 1 of Avoidant Personality Disorder) begins, "You've said that you have [*Have you*] avoided jobs or tasks that involved having to deal with a lot of people."

- If the subject circled "YES" for Question 1 on the SCID-5-SPQ, the interviewer has also circled the corresponding Question 1 (i.e., the far-left numeral "1") of the SCID-5-PD. The interviewer would then begin SCID-5-PD Question 1 as follows: "You've said that you have avoided jobs or tasks that involved having to deal with a lot of people."

- If the subject circled "NO" for Question 1 on the SCID-5-SPQ, the corresponding SCID-5-PD question is skipped and Avoidant Personality Disorder Criterion 1 is rated "0."

- If the subject circled neither "YES" nor "NO" for Question 1 on the SCID-5-SPQ (e.g., the subject did not understand the question, was unsure of his or her answer, or was too embarrassed to answer), the interviewer would ask Question 1 of the SCID-5-PD starting with the bracketed italicized text, leaving out the initial wording "You've said that you have" as follows: "Have you avoided jobs or tasks that involved having to deal with a lot of people?"

Some of the DSM-5 criteria in the SCID-5-PD have more than one left-numbered question (e.g., Criterion A1 for Schizotypal Personality Disorder, field code PD36, contains Questions 33, 34, and 35). In such cases, the criterion should be evaluated during the full SCID-5-PD interview if *any* of the corresponding SCID-5-SPQ questions have been answered "YES" or left unanswered.

Further Exploration of "NO" Answers

When the interviewer is administering the SCID-5-PD, sometimes it may be helpful to re-ask the screening questions that were answered "NO" on the SCID-5-SPQ. For example, Criterion 1 for Narcissistic Personality Disorder ("grandiose sense of self-importance") has two corresponding questions on the SCID-5-SPQ (Questions 60 and 61). If Question 60 ("Are you more important, more talented, or more successful than most other people?") is answered "NO" and Question 61 ("Have people told you that you have too high an opinion of yourself?") is answered "YES," Narcissistic Personality Disorder Criterion 1 should be explored further in the SCID-5-PD by asking the subject for examples. If there is still not enough information to decide whether to rate Criterion 1 with a "2," the interviewer should re-ask Question 60 starting with the italicized text (even though it was answered "NO" on the SCID-5-SPQ) to be absolutely sure that it is a true negative.

As discussed in Section 3.4, "Screening Personality Questionnaire," using the SCID-5-SPQ saves interview time because, in general, items circled "NO" on the questionnaire are skipped during the course of administering the SCID-5-PD interview. However, there are two circumstances in which questions that are answered "NO" on the SCID-5-SPQ (and therefore not circled on the SCID-5-PD) should be explored in the SCID-5-PD interview:

- When there is a clinical basis to suspect that the item is true. For example, even if the subject has denied all of the items for Narcissistic Personality Disorder in the SCID-5-SPQ, if during the interview the subject presents himself in a grandiose manner or acts entitled, the interviewer should ask all of the questions for Narcissistic Personality Disorder during the SCID-5-PD interview, despite the negative answers on the SCID-5-SPQ.
- When the number of Personality Disorder criteria rated "2" are only one criterion short of the required diagnostic threshold for a particular disorder. For example, if three criteria for Avoidant Personality Disorder are rated "2" (one less than the four required), all of the remaining items should be probed during the SCID-5-PD interview, even if they were denied on the SCID-5-SPQ.

4.7 Use of the SCID-5-PD Without the SCID-5-SPQ

The SCID-5-PD may be administered without the SCID-5-SPQ. This may be especially desirable in situations in which the interviewer wishes to focus on a limited number of disorders. When the SCID-5-PD is used without the SCID-5-SPQ, all of the SCID-5-PD questions should be asked, starting with the italicized phrases in brackets and omitting the initial words preceding the brackets (e.g., "You've said that..."). For example, Question 16 (Criterion 1 for Obsessive-Compulsive Personality Disorder) states, "You've said that you are [Are you] the kind of person who spends a lot of time focusing on details, order, or organization, or making lists and schedules." This should be rephrased as follows: "Are you the kind of person who spends a lot of time focusing on details, order, or organization, or making lists and schedules?"

5. SCID-5-PD Item-by-Item Commentary

This section contains commentaries for each criterion of the 10 DSM-5 Personality Disorders in the SCID-5-PD. Please refer to this section for help in interpreting the meaning of the criterion and for help in distinguishing the criterion from similar items in the other Personality Disorders. For ease of reference, each DSM-5 criterion below is followed by Interviewer's Questions, which comprise all the left-numbered SCID-5-PD interviewer questions related to each criterion.

5.1   Avoidant Personality Disorder

1. Avoids occupational activities that involve significant interpersonal contact because of fears of criticism, disapproval, or rejection.

> **Interviewer's Questions:** You've said that you have [*Have you*] avoided jobs or tasks that involved having to deal with a lot of people. Give me some examples. What was the reason that you avoided these [JOBS OR TASKS]? (Is it because you just don't like to be around people, or is it because you are afraid of being criticized or rejected?)

Commentary: Because of a fear of rejection, or of saying or doing the wrong thing, people with Avoidant Personality Disorder typically avoid jobs or school activities that put them in contact with other people (e.g., "front desk" assignments or group projects). They prefer to work by themselves and may even refuse promotions because the new position would make them more visible and, therefore, vulnerable to criticism or humiliation by others. This is in contrast to individuals with Schizotypal or Schizoid Personality Disorder, who avoid occupational activities involving significant interpersonal contact just because they do not like to be around people.

2. Is unwilling to get involved with people unless certain of being liked.

> **Interviewer's Questions:** You've said that [*Do*] you avoid making friends with people unless you are certain they will like you. Do you avoid joining in group activities unless you are sure that you will be welcomed and accepted? If you don't know whether someone likes you, would you ever make the first move?

Commentary: Many people are hesitant to initiate a social interaction because of a fear of being rejected. People with Avoidant Personality Disorder are more extreme in this regard and tend to watch from the sidelines until they are certain they will be accepted. This differs from the next criterion which involves putting limits on the intimacy of a close relationship.

3. Shows restraint within intimate relationships because of the fear of being shamed or ridiculed.

> **Interviewer's Questions:** You've said that [*Do*] you find it hard to be "open" even with people you are close to. Why is this? (Are you afraid of being made fun of or embarrassed?)

Commentary: Although able to establish intimate relationships when there is the assurance of uncritical acceptance, people with this disorder have difficulty talking about themselves and withhold intimate feelings for fear of being exposed, ridiculed, or shamed.

4. Is preoccupied with being criticized or rejected in social situations.

> **Interviewer's Questions:** You've said that *[Do]* you often worry about being criticized or rejected in social situations. Give me some examples. Do you spend a lot of time worrying about this?

Commentary: People with Avoidant or Narcissistic Personality Disorder may be hypersensitive to criticism, reacting to even minor criticisms with feelings of hurt or embarrassment. However, while individuals with Narcissistic Personality Disorder do not expect to be criticized and are surprised, indignant, and outraged when it happens, people with Avoidant Personality Disorder operate on the assumption that they will be criticized. Because most people can be hurt by especially severe criticism, it is important to establish that the amount of distress is well beyond the response of most people to similar criticism and that the person with this symptom is so constantly on guard against the possibility of being criticized that he or she spends a lot of time thinking or worrying about it.

5. Is inhibited in new interpersonal situations because of feelings of inadequacy.

> **Interviewer's Questions:** You've said that you're *[Are you]* usually quiet when you meet new people. Why is that? (Is it because you feel in some way inadequate or not good enough?)

Commentary: People with this disorder tend to be silent and "invisible," particularly in new situations, because they feel that anything they say will be "wrong" or will reveal their inadequacy.

6. Views self as socially inept, personally unappealing, or inferior to others.

> **Interviewer's Questions:** You've said that *[Do]* you believe that you're not as good, as smart, or as attractive as most other people. Tell me about that.

Commentary: The pervasive low self-esteem of people with this disorder is evident in the various ways they put themselves down. They may, unrealistically, believe that they are ugly or stupid, and that they do not know what to say in social situations or that they always do or say the wrong thing.

7. Is unusually reluctant to take personal risks or to engage in any new activities because they may prove embarrassing.

> **Interviewer's Questions:** You've said that you're *[Are you]* afraid to do things that might be challenging or to try anything new. Is that because you are afraid of being embarrassed? Give me some examples.

Commentary: In some people with Avoidant Personality Disorder, their avoidance becomes such a generalized phenomenon that they refuse to do anything outside of their normal routine or comfort zone. They may see any new project or activity only as an opportunity to reveal how inept, ugly, or otherwise unworthy they are.

They may therefore avoid job interviews, classes, or learning how to do anything new, from skiing to computer programming, for fear of doing it wrong.

5.2   Dependent Personality Disorder

1. **Has difficulty making everyday decisions without an excessive amount of advice and reassurance from others.**

> **Interviewer's Questions:** You've said that it is *[Is it]* hard for you to make everyday decisions—like what to wear or what to order in a restaurant, without advice and reassurance from others. Can you give me some examples of the kinds of decisions you would ask for advice or reassurance about? (Does this happen most of the time?)

Commentary: People with Dependent Personality Disorder need others to make decisions for them. This criterion refers to an inability to make everyday decisions (e.g., deciding which clothes to wear in the morning, making a selection from a menu) rather than major decisions (e.g., whether to get married, where to live), which is covered in Criterion 2. This personality trait must be differentiated from indecisiveness (a feature of Major Depressive Episode), in which the primary pathology is an inability to make decisions rather than the need to rely on others for help in making them.

2. **Needs others to assume responsibility for most major areas of his or her life.**

> **Interviewer's Questions:** You've said that you *[Do you]* depend on other people to handle important areas of your life, such as finances, child care, or living arrangements. Give me some examples. (Is this more than just getting advice from people?) (Has this happened with MOST important areas of your life?)

Commentary: People with Dependent Personality Disorder typically allow and even encourage others to assume responsibility for most of the major areas of their life. Adults with this disorder typically depend on a parent or spouse to decide where they should live, what kind of job they should have, and which neighbors to befriend. Adolescents with this disorder may allow their parent(s) to decide with whom they should associate, how they should spend their free time, and what school or college they should attend. Seeking advice about such decisions is normal and by itself does not constitute sufficient evidence to warrant a rating of "2" on this criterion. For a rating of "2" to be justified, the person must clearly defer the decisions to other people. Use careful clinical judgment when considering this question for adolescents and young adults, making allowances for age-appropriate dependence on parents or parental surrogates. Also be sure to consider subcultural norms in rating this criterion (e.g., arranged marriages). Dependent Personality Disorder may occur in an individual who has a serious medical condition or disability, but in such cases the difficulty in taking responsibility must go beyond what would normally be associated with that condition or disability.

3. **Has difficulty expressing disagreement with others because of fear of loss of support or approval. (Note: Do not include realistic fears of retribution.)**

> **Interviewer's Questions:** You've said that *[Do]* you have trouble disagreeing with people even when you think they are wrong. Give me some examples of when that has happened. What are you afraid would happen if you disagree?

Commentary: Passivity and subjugation are often characteristic features of Dependent Personality Disorder, and may be manifested by the person being excessively agreeable, for fear of losing others' support or approval. Individuals with Dependent Personality Disorder feel so unable to function alone that they will agree with things that they feel are wrong rather than risk losing the help of those to whom they look for guidance. Moreover, they do not get appropriately angry at others whose support and nurturance they need for fear of alienating them. In order to warrant a rating of "2," this behavior should not be limited to interactions with people of a higher rank or status (e.g., bosses, professors), and should not be rated "2" if the individual's concerns regarding the consequences of expressing disagreement are realistic (e.g., realistic fears of retribution from an abusive spouse).

4. **Has difficulty initiating projects or doing things on his or her own (because of a lack of self-confidence in judgment or abilities rather than a lack of motivation or energy).**

> **Interviewer's Questions:** You've said *[Do]* you find it hard to start projects or do things on your own. Give me some examples. Why is that? (Is this because you are not sure you can do it right?) (Can you do it as long as there is someone there to help you?)

Commentary: Because of their excessive need for the advice and support of others, people with Dependent Personality Disorder avoid working on their own or taking the initiative in starting projects or tasks, and prefer to depend on others. Evidence supporting a rating of "2" should be restricted to tasks that can ordinarily be done without the help of other people. Be sure to establish that this overreliance on others is not limited to periods of depression.

5. **Goes to excessive lengths to obtain nurturance and support from others, to the point of volunteering to do things that are unpleasant.**

> **Interviewer's Questions:** You've said that it is *[Is it]* so important to you to be taken care of by others that you are willing to do unpleasant or unreasonable things for them. Give me some examples of these kinds of things.

Commentary: People with Dependent Personality Disorder typically subjugate their own needs to the needs of others in order to get their nurturance and support. They are willing to submit to what others want, even if the demands are unreasonable. Their need to maintain a bond will often result in imbalanced or distorted relationships. They may make extraordinary self-sacrifices or tolerate verbal, physical, or sexual abuse. Individuals with Borderline Personality Disorder may also subjugate their needs to those with whom they are in a relationship, but this is motivated by a fear of abandonment rather than an excessive need for nurturance and support.

6. **Feels uncomfortable or helpless when alone because of exaggerated fears of being unable to care for himself or herself.**

> **Interviewer's Questions:** You've said that *[Do]* you usually feel uncomfortable when you are by yourself. Why is that? (Is it because you need someone to take care of you?)

Commentary: Individuals with Dependent Personality Disorder will often "tag along" with important others just to avoid being alone, even if they are not interested or involved in what is happening. In some severe cases of Dependent Personality Disorder, the dependence on others becomes so extreme that the person experiences distress when alone even for a few hours, and will therefore go to great lengths to avoid being alone. When forced to be alone, he or she may make repeated urgent phone calls to "caretakers." Note that people with Borderline Personality Disorder can also become distressed when alone. However, in Dependent Personality Disorder, the person's primary concern is that he or she does not have the requisite skills to take care of himself or herself, whereas in Borderline Personality Disorder, the concern is that the person will "fall apart" if he or she is alone.

7. **Urgently seeks another relationship as a source of care and support when a close relationship ends.**

> **Interviewer's Questions:** You've said that when a close relationship ends, you *[When a close relationship ends, do you]* feel you immediately have to find someone else to take care of you. Tell me about that. (Have you reacted this way most of the time when close relationships have ended?)

Commentary: Although most people feel upset when a close relationship ends, people with Dependent Personality Disorder are overwhelmed by the loss, and often urgently seek an immediate replacement for the lost person. They may become quickly attached to another person because they feel unable to care for themselves. An inability to function in the context of a stressful life events such as the breakup of a relationship or the death of a loved one is not sufficient to justify a rating of "2" for this criterion.

8. **Is unrealistically preoccupied with fears of being left to take care of himself or herself.**

> **Interviewer's Questions:** You've said that *[Do]* you worry a lot about being left alone to take care of yourself. What makes you think that you are going to be left alone to take care of yourself? (How realistic is this fear?) How much do you worry about this?

Commentary: People with Dependent Personality Disorder often become preoccupied with the fear of being abandoned because of their feeling that they cannot cope by themselves, even when there is no real threat of abandonment. This criterion should not be rated "2" if the supporting evidence is limited to particular circumstances, such as the impending death of a loved one, or if the fear of abandonment is a realistic concern (e.g., an elderly person with no surviving friends or family, a person with a disabling physical illness).

5.3 Obsessive-Compulsive Personality Disorder

1. **Is preoccupied with details, rules, lists, order, organization, or schedules to the extent that the major point of the activity is lost.**

    Interviewer's Questions: You've said that you are *[Are you]* the kind of person who spends a lot of time focusing on details, order, or organization, or making lists and schedules. Tell me about that. Do you spend so much time doing this that the point of what you were trying to do gets lost? (For example, you spend so much time preparing a list of things you have to do that you don't have enough time to get them done.)

    Commentary: People with Obsessive-Compulsive Personality Disorder are overly concerned with the details, process, or method of accomplishing a task. When this is extreme, so much time is spent focusing on these details that they become ends in themselves and the task is prolonged, only partially completed, or not completed at all. For example, when such individuals misplace a list of things to be done, they will spend an inordinate amount of time looking for the list rather than spending a few moments re-creating it from memory and proceeding to accomplish the tasks. While this is usually most relevant in occupational situations (e.g., with projects at work) or housework, it may occur in other settings, such as becoming so preoccupied with planning the minute details of a trip that the person is unable to enjoy the trip itself.

2. **Shows perfectionism that interferes with task completion (e.g., is unable to complete a project because his or her own overly strict standards are not met).**

    Interviewer's Questions: You've said that *[Do]* you have trouble finishing things because you spend so much time trying to get them exactly right. Give me some examples. (How often does this happen?)

    Commentary: Individuals with Obsessive-Compulsive Personality Disorder may become so involved in making every detail of a project absolutely perfect that the project is never finished. For example, the completion of a paper for school is delayed by numerous time-consuming rewrites that all come up short of "perfection."

    Perfectionism is a trait that can result in occupational productivity and success. This criterion should be rated "2" only if there is evidence that the perfectionism is so pronounced that it interferes with task completion; tasks are never completed or are significantly delayed because of the insistence on getting things exactly right, or they take an inordinately lengthy amount of time to complete. This criterion differs from Criterion 1 in that the impairment in functioning is due to perfectionism rather than (or in addition to) getting lost in the details.

3. **Is excessively devoted to work and productivity to the exclusion of leisure activities and friendships (not accounted for by obvious economic necessity).**

> **Interviewer's Questions:** You've said that you are *[Are you]* very devoted to your work or to being productive. Are you so devoted that you rarely get to spend time with friends, go on vacation, or do things just for fun? (When you do take time off, do you always take work along because you can't stand to "waste time"?)

Commentary: This criterion should be rated "2" if the person is so dedicated to his or her work that there is virtually no time left for the pursuit of leisure activities (e.g., has no hobbies; never attends sports, concerts, movies) or interpersonal relationships (e.g., rarely spends time with spouse or children or socializing with friends). The person may provide rationalizations for this behavior (e.g., "I love my work," "it's important so I can get ahead," "I can't get all my work done during the day"), but the only explanations that should result in a rating of "0" are those involving obvious economic necessity (e.g., working a second job to provide basic support for family) or special short-term circumstances (e.g., a brief period of long work hours before a deadline; a medical internship).

4. **Is overconscientious, scrupulous, and inflexible about matters of morality, ethics, or values (not accounted for by cultural or religious identification).**

> **Interviewer's Questions:** You've said that *[Do]* you have very high standards about what is right and what is wrong. Give me some examples of your high standards. (Do you follow rules to the letter of the law, no matter what? Do you insist that others also follow the rules? Can you give me some examples?) *IF GIVES RELIGIOUS EXAMPLE:* Are you stricter than other people who share your religious views?

Commentary: This question concerns the tendency of people with Obsessive-Compulsive Personality Disorder to extend their inflexible nature and concern with high standards to the arena of morality and ethics. Many people believe they have higher moral standards than others. This criterion should be rated "2" only if there is evidence that the person is overly conscientious, rigid, scrupulous, or self-righteous. Such individuals have an excessive concern about doing what is right and may be very worried about having done something wrong. Individuals with this disorder tend to be rigidly deferential to authority and rules and insist on quite literal compliance, with no rule bending for extenuating circumstances. It is important to consider the cultural and religious context of the person because this behavior often appears in a religious context; the criterion should be rated "2" only if the person is considerably more inflexible or conscientious than others of the same religious or cultural background. An example would be someone who chastises friends for engaging in harmless gossip.

5. **Is unable to discard worn-out or worthless objects even when they have no sentimental value.**

> **Interviewer's Questions:** You've said that *[Do]* you have trouble throwing things out because they might come in handy someday. Give me some examples of things that you're unable to throw out. (What about things that are worn out or worthless?)

Commentary: Often these individuals will admit to being "pack rats." They regard discarding objects as wasteful because "you never know when you might need something" and will become upset if someone tries to get rid of the things they have saved. People with this trait save things that they are extremely unlikely to use again (e.g., numerous plastic containers or corks, many years' worth of newspapers and magazines). Because it is so common for people to save things in case they are needed in the future, this criterion should be rated "2" only if the behavior is clearly pathological. If the person only has difficulty throwing away things that have some special personal importance (e.g., classroom notes from junior high school), then this is not evidence that the trait is present.

6. **Is reluctant to delegate tasks or to work with others unless they submit to exactly his or her way of doing things.**

> **Interviewer's Questions:** You've said that it is *[Is it]* hard for you to work with other people or ask others to do things if they don't agree to do things exactly the way you want. Tell me about that. (Does this happen often?) (Do you often end up doing things yourself to make sure they are done right?)

Commentary: People with Obsessive-Compulsive Personality Disorder characteristically insist that things always be done their way. Because of extensive use of rationalization, it may be difficult to establish that the person's insistence is truly "unreasonable"; the person may provide plausible explanations that lend credence to the contention that his or her way is indeed the best. In these cases, evidence should be culled from the person's stubbornness in activities in which the "best way" is debatable, such as household cleaning tasks. Often there will have been complaints from others about the person's bossiness, and frequently a person with this characteristic ends up doing such tasks himself or herself in order to be sure they are done the "right" way.

7. **Adopts a miserly spending style toward both self and others; money is viewed as something to be hoarded for future catastrophes.**

> **Interviewer's Questions:** You've said that it is *[Is it]* hard for you to spend money on yourself and other people. Why? (Is this because you're worried about not having enough in the future when you might really need it? What might you need it for?) Has anyone said that you are "stingy" or "miserly"?

Commentary: Individuals with Obsessive-Compulsive Personality Disorder often maintain a standard of living far below what they can afford, believing that spending must be tightly controlled to provide for future catastrophes. The personality trait of generosity is on a continuum, ranging from self-sacrificing to stingy. This criterion should be rated "2" only if the person is clearly much less generous than most others would be in comparable circumstances.

8. Shows rigidity and stubbornness.

Interviewer's Questions: You've said that once you've made plans, it is *[Once you've made plans, is it]* hard for you to make changes. Tell me about that. (Are you so concerned about having things done the one "correct" way that you have trouble going along with anyone else's ideas? Tell me about that.) You've said that other people have *[Have other people]* said that you are stubborn. Tell me about that.

Commentary: Individuals with Obsessive-Compulsive Personality Disorder are so concerned about having things done the one "correct" way that they have trouble going along with anyone else's ideas. These individuals typically plan ahead in meticulous detail and are unwilling to consider changes. Even when they recognize that it may be in their best interest to compromise, they may stubbornly refuse to do so, arguing that it is "the principle of the thing."

5.4 Paranoid Personality Disorder

A1. Suspects, without sufficient basis, that others are exploiting, harming, or deceiving him or her.

Interviewer's Questions: You've said that *[Do]* you often get the feeling that people are using you, hurting you, or lying to you. What makes you think that?

Commentary: This item expresses the core feature of the disorder, namely, a fundamental expectation that others will exploit, take advantage of, or hurt the person. When trying to make an assessment of this criterion, the focus should be on evaluating a general paranoid orientation, in addition to looking for specific examples of paranoid ideation. In cases in which the paranoid ideation reaches delusional proportions, a diagnosis of a Psychotic Disorder should be seriously considered.

A2. Is preoccupied with unjustified doubts about the loyalty or trustworthiness of friends or associates.

Interviewer's Questions: You've said that you are *[Are you]* a very private person who rarely confides in other people. Is it because you don't trust your friends or the people you work with? Why don't you trust them? Do you spend a lot of time thinking about this?

Commentary: Because it is often very difficult to determine whether a lack of trust is unjustified in a particular case, this criterion should be rated "2" only if the person is preoccupied with these kinds of doubts in almost all relationships. This criterion differs from Criterion 1, in that Criterion 1 reflects a general paranoid perspective about the environment, whereas this criterion reflects the person's expectations of betrayal even by family, friends, or coworkers.

A3. Is reluctant to confide in others because of unwarranted fear that the information will be used maliciously against him or her.

Interviewer's Questions: You've said that *[Do]* you find that it is best not to let other people know much about you because they will use it against you. When has this happened? Tell me about that.

Commentary: It is important to determine that the reason for being reluctant to confide in others is a fear of some harm resulting from having confided the information, rather than merely a fear of rejection (which is characteristic of Avoidant Personality Disorder). In addition, this criterion should not be rated "2" if the reluctance to confide in a particular person seems justified based on previous experience with that person.

A4. Reads hidden demeaning or threatening meanings into benign remarks or events.

Interviewer's Questions: You've said that *[Do]* you often feel that people are threatening or insulting you by the things they say or do. Tell me about that.

Commentary: This characteristic consists of idiosyncratic personalized interpretations of innocuous behavior as having a malevolent intent. This is the "paranoid" version of Criterion A1 in Schizotypal Personality Disorder, in which an event or object in the person's environment is perceived to have a particular or unusual significance (i.e., an idea of reference). For a "2" rating of this criterion for Paranoid Personality Disorder, the ideas of reference must have a threatening or demeaning content. Note that the interview question does not directly inquire whether the subject reads hidden demeaning or threatening meanings into benign remarks. Once the subject describes having the feeling that people are threatening or insulting him or her by the things they say or do, the interviewer needs to 1) find out exactly what the subject believes people are saying or doing that feels threatening or demeaning and then 2) decide whether the subject is finding hidden threats in what people say or do, as opposed to picking up overt threats.

A5. Persistently bears grudges (i.e., is unforgiving of insults, injuries, or slights).

Interviewer's Questions: You've said that you're *[Are you]* the kind of person who holds grudges or takes a long time to forgive people who have insulted or slighted you. Tell me about that. You've said that there are *[Are there]* a lot of people you can't forgive because they did or said something to you a long time ago. Tell me about that.

Commentary: To qualify as a "grudge," the person's reaction must be clearly out of proportion to the severity or intensity of the insult or injury. For example, a lifelong grudge against a person for murdering a friend would not be out of proportion, but refusal to speak to a close friend for several years after a minor argument would be.

A6. Perceives attacks on his or her character or reputation that are not apparent to others and is quick to react angrily or to counterattack.

> **Interviewer's Questions:** You've said that *[Do]* you often get angry or lash out when someone criticizes or insults you in some way. Give me some examples. (Do others say that you often take offense too easily?)

Commentary: There are two parts to this criterion. First, the person must be hypersensitive to minor insults, indignities, or omissions. Second (and distinguishing this criterion from the Avoidant Personality Disorder "easily hurt by criticism" criterion), the person is quick to react with anger or counterattack.

A7. Has recurrent suspicions, without justification, regarding fidelity of spouse or sexual partner.

> **Interviewer's Questions:** You've said that you have *[Have you]* sometimes suspected that your spouse or partner has been unfaithful. Tell me about that. (What clues did you have? What did you do about it? Were you right?)

Commentary: The usual difficulty in assessing this criterion is determining whether or not the jealousy is "pathological" (i.e., persistent and unjustified). This often requires careful questioning or establishing frequent instances of jealousy occurring in several different relationships. There is often excessive and inappropriate behavior associated with the jealousy, such as neglecting other responsibilities in order to monitor a spouse's (or lover's) activities.

B. Does not occur exclusively during the course of Schizophrenia, a Bipolar Disorder or Depressive Disorder With Psychotic Features, or another Psychotic Disorder and is not attributable to the physiological effects of another medical condition.

> **Interviewer's Questions:** *IF THERE IS EVIDENCE OF A PSYCHOTIC DISORDER:* Does this happen only when you are having (SXS OF DISORDER)? *IF THERE IS EVIDENCE OF PROLONGED EXCESSIVE ALCOHOL OR DRUG USE THAT RESULTS IN SYMPTOMS THAT RESEMBLE PARANOID PD:* Does this happen only when you are drunk or high or withdrawing from alcohol or drugs? *IF THERE IS EVIDENCE OF A GMC THAT CAUSES SYMPTOMS THAT RESEMBLE PARANOID PD:* Were you like that before (ONSET OF GMC)?

Commentary: Paranoid symptoms can occur as a result of substance use (e.g., cocaine intoxication) or a medical condition (e.g., Alzheimer's disease, Parkinson's disease). If the paranoid ideation is confined to periods of substance intoxication or withdrawal or if it occurs only during a GMC that is known to cause such symptoms, Paranoid Personality Disorder should not be diagnosed. Moreover, a number of Psychotic Disorders (e.g., Delusional Disorder, Schizophrenia, Bipolar and Depressive Disorders With Psychotic Features) are characterized by paranoid ideation that may reach delusional proportions. If the paranoid symptoms occur exclusively during the course of a Psychotic Disorder, Paranoid Personality Disorder should not also be diagnosed.

5.5 Schizotypal Personality Disorder

A1. Ideas of reference (excluding delusions of reference).

> **Interviewer's Questions:** You've said that when you are out in public and see people talking, *[When you are out in public and see people talking, do]* you often feel that they are talking about you. Tell me more about this. You've said that when you are around people, you *[When you are around people, do you]* often get the feeling that you are being watched or stared at. Tell me more about this. You've said that you *[Do you]* often get the feeling that the words to a song or something in a movie or on TV has a special meaning for you in particular. Tell me more about this.

Commentary: Ideas of reference (also known as referential thinking) are typical of the ideation that is characteristic of Schizotypal Personality Disorder. A person with an idea of reference has the belief that an event, object, or other person in the immediate environment has a particular or unusual significance to him or her. A common example is a person who often has the feeling that when he sees a group of strangers talking to each other, they are really talking about him. Much less common is the person who believes objects in the environment, such as the words to a song or something on the TV or radio, contain a special message for him or her. For example, a woman waking up in the morning to the Beatles song "Let it Be" on the radio believes that this is a message to her that she is supposed to forgive her parents for the way they treated her when she was a little girl. An idea of reference should be distinguished from a delusion of reference, in which the referential idea is held with delusional intensity (i.e., the person firmly believes that the delusion of reference is true and will not seriously entertain alternative explanations). In cases in which the referential thinking reaches delusional proportions, a diagnosis of a Psychotic Disorder should be seriously considered.

A2. Odd beliefs or magical thinking that influences behavior and is inconsistent with subcultural norms (e.g., superstitiousness, belief in clairvoyance, telepathy, or "sixth sense"; in children and adolescents, bizarre fantasies or preoccupations).

> **Interviewer's Questions:** You've said that you are *[Are you]* a superstitious person. What are some of your superstitions? How have they affected what you say or do? Do you know other people who do these things? You've said that you have *[Have you ever]* felt that you could make things happen just by making a wish or thinking about them. Tell me about that. (How did it affect you?) You've said that you have *[Have*

you] had personal experiences with the supernatural. Tell me about that. (How did it affect you?) You've said that you [*Do you*] believe that you have a "sixth sense" that allows you to know and predict things. Tell me about that. (How does it affect you?)

Commentary: Some superstitions and other beliefs that are inconsistent with the laws of nature and physics are common in most societies and cultures. To fulfill a "2" rating for this criterion, the person must do more than just acknowledge having such beliefs; he or she must report some influence of these beliefs on his or her behavior. For example, a person who reports only believing in the existence of extrasensory perception (ESP) would not receive a "2" rating on this criterion; instead, the person must also report a personal experience with ESP that influenced his or her behavior. In addition, a "2" rating should be considered only for beliefs that deviate considerably from the norms of the person's subculture. *Magical thinking* is a particular kind of "odd belief" in which the person believes that his or her words, thoughts, or actions will cause something to occur or prevent something from occurring in a way that violates the physical laws of cause and effect. An example is a person believing that his intense wish to win the lottery was responsible for his winning. Odd beliefs and magical thinking should be distinguished from similar beliefs held with delusional intensity (e.g., the person firmly believes that he can read other people's minds or that he has the power to make things happen simply by thinking about them and will not seriously entertain alternative explanations). In cases in which the odd beliefs reach delusional proportions, a diagnosis of a Psychotic Disorder should be seriously considered.

A3. Unusual perceptual experiences, including bodily illusions.

Interviewer's Questions: You've said that you [*Do you*] often have the feeling that everything is unreal, that you are detached from your body or mind, or that you are an outside observer of your own thoughts or movements. Give me some examples. (Were you drinking or taking drugs at the time?) You've said that [*Do*] you often see things that other people don't see. Give me some examples. (Were you drinking or taking drugs at the time?) You've said that you [*Do you*] often hear a voice softly speaking your name. Tell me more about that. (Were you drinking or taking drugs at the time?) You've said that you have [*Have you*] had the sense that some person or force is around you, even though you cannot see anyone. Tell me more about that. (Were you drinking or taking drugs at the time?)

Commentary: Unusual perceptual experiences should be distinguished from psychotic hallucinations (i.e., abnormal perceptual experiences that are persistent, believed by the individual to be real rather than a product of his or her own mind, and that are of sufficient intensity to have an impact on the person's behavior). In cases in which the hallucinations are sufficiently severe to be considered evidence of psychosis, a diagnosis of a Psychotic Disorder should be seriously considered. In addition, unusual perceptual experiences that are due to drugs (e.g., hallucinogens), physical disorders (e.g., metabolic encephalopathy), or natural phenomena (e.g., hypnagogic or hypnopompic hallucinations that occur upon falling asleep or awakening from sleep) should not be considered evidence for making a rating of "2" for this criterion.

A4. Odd thinking and speech (e.g., vague, circumstantial, metaphorical, overelaborate, or stereotyped).

OBSERVED DURING INTERVIEW

Commentary: This criterion is rated on the basis of the interviewer's observation. Other examples of odd speech include idiosyncratic word usage; neologisms; speech with no content; and stilted, overly metaphorical, overly concrete, or overly tangential and circumstantial speech. Note that speech that is so disordered as to be classifiable as "loosening of associations" or "incoherence" suggests a diagnosis of Schizophrenia.

A5. Suspiciousness or paranoid ideation.

Commentary: This criterion can be rated "2" if any of Paranoid Personality Disorder Criteria A1, A2, A3, A4, or A7 have been rated "2." The relevant criteria in Paranoid Personality Disorder are as follows:

- Criterion A1: Suspects, without sufficient basis, that others are exploiting, harming, or deceiving him or her.
- Criterion A2: Is preoccupied with unjustified doubts about the loyalty or trustworthiness of friends or associates.
- Criterion A3: Is reluctant to confide in others because of unwarranted fear that the information will be used maliciously against him or her.
- Criterion A4: Reads hidden demeaning or threatening meanings into benign remarks or events.
- Criterion A7: Has recurrent suspicions, without justification, regarding fidelity of spouse or sexual partner.

If the interviewer has chosen to skip the assessment of Paranoid Personality Disorder in the SCID-5-PD, Criterion A5 can be rated "2" provided that there is clinical evidence that the subject is generally suspicious of other people or exhibits persistent paranoid ideation.

A6. Inappropriate or constricted affect.

OBSERVED DURING INTERVIEW

Commentary: This criterion is rated on the basis of the interviewer's observation, as well as any other information that is available. Inappropriate affect is defined as an incongruity between the content of what the person is saying and his or her vocal inflections and facial expression. It is often expressed as inappropriate cheerfulness (e.g., smiling brightly when telling about something terrible that happened). Do not include inappropriate laughter that is due to anxiety. Evidence for constricted affect includes unchanging facial expression, monotonous or unvarying vocal inflection, absence of expressive gestures, keeping a rigid posture, and poor eye contact. Any evidence of constricted affect must be present over a prolonged period of time and should clearly not be due to depressed mood or medication side effects (e.g., neuroleptics).

A7. Behavior or appearance that is odd, eccentric, or peculiar.

OBSERVED DURING INTERVIEW

Commentary: This criterion is rated on the basis of the interviewer's observation, as well as any other information that is available from informants. Examples of odd behavior should be present over a prolonged period of time and not due to some other mental disorder (e.g., Manic Episode, Schizophrenia). Examples would include a person who can be seen talking to himself in the street, a person who wears items of clothing that obviously do not fit together, or wearing many layers of clothing on a warm day. This criterion is not, however, meant to apply to individuals who dress in an unusual way simply to be stylish.

A8. Lack of close friends or confidants other than first-degree relatives.

Interviewer's Questions: You've said that there are *[Are there]* very few people who you're really close to outside of your immediate family. How many close friends do you have?

Commentary: People with Schizoid or Schizotypal Personality Disorder typically have very few friends or confidants because they tend to avoid close relationships with other people, albeit for different reasons. People with Schizoid Personality Disorder avoid close friendships because they have little interest in relationships with other people. Those with Schizotypal Personality Disorder feel uncomfortable in relationships because of excessive social anxiety and social awkwardness and therefore avoid them.

A9. Excessive social anxiety that does not diminish with familiarity and tends to be associated with paranoid fears rather than negative judgments about self.

Interviewer's Questions: You've said that *[Do]* you often feel nervous when you are around people you don't know very well. What are you nervous about? Is it because you are worried about being taken advantage of or hurt in some way rather than being rejected or criticized? (Are you still anxious even after you've known them for a while?)

Commentary: A rating of "2" for this criterion requires that the person be much more uncomfortable than most people are in social situations, even with familiar people. The social anxiety in Schizotypal Personality Disorder is rooted in a fundamental inability to relate to other people and is associated with paranoid fears. For this reason, familiarity does not provide reassurance and comfort. In contrast, in Avoidant Personality Disorder, familiarity reduces anxiety because it alleviates fear of humiliation and rejection, which is most relevant in the initial stages of a relationship.

B. Does not occur exclusively during the course of Schizophrenia, a Bipolar Disorder or Depressive Disorder With Psychotic Features, another Psychotic Disorder, or Autism Spectrum Disorder.

> **Interviewer's Questions:** *IF THERE IS EVIDENCE OF A PSYCHOTIC DISORDER:* Does this happen only when you are having (SXS OF PSYCHOTIC DISORDER)? *IF THERE IS EVIDENCE OF PROLONGED EXCESSIVE ALCOHOL OR DRUG USE THAT RESULTS IN SYMPTOMS THAT RESEMBLE SCHIZOTYPAL PD:* Does this happen only when you are drunk or high or withdrawing from alcohol or drugs? *IF THERE IS EVIDENCE OF A GMC THAT CAUSES SYMPTOMS THAT RESEMBLE SCHIZOTYPAL PD:* Were you like that before (ONSET OF GMC)?

Commentary: Paranoid symptoms, unusual perceptual experiences, and odd beliefs can occur as a result of substance use (e.g., cocaine intoxication) or a medical condition (e.g., Alzheimer's disease). If the symptoms suggestive of Schizotypal Personality Disorder are confined to periods of substance intoxication or withdrawal or occur exclusively during a GMC that causes such symptoms, Schizotypal Personality Disorder should not be diagnosed. Moreover, a number of Psychotic Disorders (e.g., Delusional Disorder, Schizophrenia, Bipolar and Depressive Disorders With Psychotic Features) are characterized by symptoms suggestive of Schizotypal Personality Disorder that at times may reach delusional proportions. If the symptoms occur exclusively during the course of a Psychotic Disorder, Schizotypal Personality Disorder should not also be diagnosed. Finally, social anxiety, lack of close friends, and odd beliefs and behavior are typical of individuals with Autism Spectrum Disorder. Schizotypal Personality Disorder should not be diagnosed in individuals with Autism Spectrum Disorder.

5.6 Schizoid Personality Disorder

A1. Neither desires nor enjoys close relationships, including being part of a family.

> **Interviewer's Questions:** You've said that it is *[Is it]* NOT important to you to have friends or romantic relationships or to be involved with your family. Tell me more about that.

Commentary: This lack of strong desire for relationships is the hallmark of Schizoid Personality Disorder and is what differentiates it from Avoidant Personality Disorder. In Avoidant Personality Disorder, the person desires close relationships but lacks them due to excessive social anxiety.

A2. Almost always chooses solitary activities.

Interviewer's Questions: You've said that you would *[Would you]* almost always rather do things alone than with other people. (Is that true both at work and during your free time?)

Commentary: Because the person with this disorder has little desire for relationships or to be around other people, it follows that he or she would almost always choose solitary activities rather than activities that involve other people. This preference should be pervasive and extend to both work and leisure activities.

A3. Has little, if any, interest in having sexual experiences with another person.

Interviewer's Questions: You've said that *[Do]* you have little or no interest in having sexual experiences with another person. Tell me more about that.

Commentary: The lack of desire to have sexual experiences with another person must have been present since adolescence and should not be due simply to a fear of rejection.

A4. Takes pleasure in few, if any, activities.

Interviewer's Questions: You've said that there are *[Are there]* really very few things that give you pleasure. Tell me about that. (What about physical things like eating a good meal or having sex?)

Commentary: Although some people with this disorder may derive pleasure from solitary intellectual activities (e.g., stamp collecting, doing mathematical problems), they generally lack the ability to take pleasure in interpersonal activities or sensory experiences (e.g., eating, sex).

A5. Lacks close friends or confidants other than first-degree relatives.

Interviewer's Questions: *PREVIOUSLY RATED IN* **CRITERION A8** *FOR SCHIZO-TYPAL PD. IF NOT PREVIOUSLY RATED THERE, USE THE FOLLOWING QUES-TION, CORRESPONDING TO* **QUESTION 44** *ON THE SCID-5-SPQ.* You've said that there are *[Are there]* very few people who you're really close to outside of your immediate family. How many close friends do you have?

Commentary: If the interviewer has already assessed the criteria for Schizotypal Personality Disorder, this criterion can be rated based on the rating for Criterion A8 (Question 44) in Schizotypal Personality Disorder. If, however, the interviewer has chosen to skip the assessment of Schizotypal Personality Disorder, the questions are provided for Criterion A5 in Schizoid Personality Disorder and should be asked here (i.e., "Are there very few people who you're really close to outside of your immediate family? How many close friends do you have?"). See the commentary for Schizotypal Personality Disorder, Criterion A8, for more guidance on making a rating of "2" for Schizoid Personality Disorder, Criterion A5.

A6. Appears indifferent to the praise or criticism of others.

> **Interviewer's Questions:** You've said that it doesn't *[Does it not]* matter to you what people think of you. How do you feel when people praise you or criticize you?

Commentary: People with this trait have little interest in relationships with other people and therefore do not care what other people think about them.

A7. Shows emotional coldness, detachment, or flattened affectivity.

> **Interviewer's Questions:** You've said that *[Do]* you rarely have strong feelings, like being very angry or feeling joyful. Tell me more about that. *ALSO CONSIDER BEHAVIOR DURING INTERVIEW*

Commentary: Behavior that can be directly observed should be the primary basis for rating this criterion. People with this trait usually display a "bland" exterior without visible emotional reactivity, speak in a monotonous tone without varying their vocal inflection, and rarely reciprocate gestures or facial expressions, such as smiles or nods. They may be oblivious to the normal subtleties of social interaction and often do not respond appropriately to social cues, so that they seem socially inept or superficial and self-absorbed. It is important to ascertain that the person characteristically appears this way (either by asking the person directly or by checking with other informants) and that this constricted affect is not due to depressed mood or to the effects of medication (e.g., neuroleptics).

B. Does not occur exclusively during the course of Schizophrenia, a Bipolar Disorder or Depressive Disorder With Psychotic Features, another Psychotic Disorder, or Autism Spectrum Disorder and is not attributable to the physiological effects of another medical condition.

> **Interviewer's Questions:** *IF THERE IS EVIDENCE OF A PSYCHOTIC DISORDER:* Does this happen only when you are having (SXS OF PSYCHOTIC DISORDER)? *IF THERE IS EVIDENCE OF PROLONGED EXCESSIVE ALCOHOL OR DRUG USE THAT RESULTS IN SYMPTOMS THAT RESEMBLE SCHIZOID PD:* Does this happen only when you are drunk or high or withdrawing from alcohol or drugs? *IF THERE IS EVIDENCE OF A GMC THAT CAUSES SYMPTOMS THAT RESEMBLE SCHIZOID PD:* Were you like that before (ONSET OF GMC)?

Commentary: Social aloofness and anhedonia can occur as a result of certain medical conditions (e.g., Alzheimer's disease, Parkinson's disease). If the symptoms suggestive of Schizoid Personality Disorder are caused by a medical condition, then a diagnosis of Personality Change Due to Another Medical Condition should be considered instead of Schizoid Personality Disorder. Moreover, a number of Psychotic Disorders (e.g., Schizophrenia, Bipolar and Depressive Disorders With Psychotic Features) can be characterized by symptoms such as social aloofness and anhedonia. If the symptoms occur exclusively during the course of a Psychotic Disorder, Schizoid Personality Disorder should not also be diagnosed. Finally, Schizoid Personality Disorder should not be diagnosed in individuals with Autism Spectrum Disorder.

5.7 Histrionic Personality Disorder

1. Is uncomfortable in situations in which he or she is not the center of attention.

> **Interviewer's Questions:** You've said that *[Do]* you like being the center of attention. How do you feel when you're not? (Uncomfortable?)

Commentary: The desire to be noticed and have other people pay attention is normal. In Histrionic Personality Disorder, this desire for attention is so extreme that it becomes insatiable. Because the person feels uncomfortable when not the center of attention, he or she will go to great lengths to insure being and remaining at the center, such as monopolizing conversations in a group of people, flamboyantly dramatizing story after story, or "making a scene."

2. Interaction with others is often characterized by inappropriate sexually seductive or provocative behavior.

> **Interviewer's Questions:** You've said that *[Do]* you tend to flirt a lot. Has anyone complained about this? *ALSO CONSIDER BEHAVIOR DURING INTERVIEW* You've said that you *[Do you]* often find yourself "coming on" to people. Tell me about that. *ALSO CONSIDER BEHAVIOR DURING INTERVIEW*

Commentary: This criterion should be rated "2" if there are striking examples of seductive behavior that is compulsive or indiscriminate (i.e., at times or in situations not related to dating, courtship, and romance). An example is someone who is flirtatious with waiters or waitresses, grocery clerks, delivery people, and so forth.

3. Displays rapidly shifting and shallow expression of emotions.

OBSERVED DURING INTERVIEW

Commentary: This observed criterion refers to rapid shifts in expressed mood that reflect the fundamental superficiality of the affect. For example, the person might get very excited about something or someone and then quickly lose interest, or throw a temper tantrum that immediately dissipates when the person's attention shifts to something else. The person's emotions are turned on and off so quickly that others may accuse the person of faking the feelings. This criterion for Histrionic Personality Disorder is distinguished from Criterion 6 of Borderline Personality Disorder ("affective instability"), in that the shifting emotions in Borderline Personality Disorder are deeper and more sustained (i.e., lasting for hours or days).

4. Consistently uses physical appearance to draw attention to self.

Interviewer's Questions: You've said that you [*Do you*] like to draw attention to yourself by the way you dress or look. Describe what you do. Do you do that kind of thing most of the time?

Commentary: Individuals with Histrionic Personality Disorder are overly concerned with impressing others by their appearance and expend an excessive amount of time, energy, and money on clothes and grooming. They may "fish for compliments" regarding appearance and may be easily and excessively upset by a critical comment about how they look or by a photograph that they regard as unflattering.

5. Has a style of speech that is excessively impressionistic and lacking in detail.

OBSERVED DURING INTERVIEW

Commentary: This criterion is rated based on the interviewer's observation. Going along with the overly dramatic presentation of the person with Histrionic Personality Disorder is a dramatic style of speech that is excessively impressionistic and is characterized by the frequent use of broad, sweeping, global statements, lacking in detail. For example, the person may describe someone as "horrible" or "wonderful" without being able to provide any supporting facts or details.

6. Shows self-dramatization, theatricality, and exaggerated expression of emotion.

Interviewer's Questions: You've said that you [*Do you*] tend to be very dramatic in your actions and speech. Tell me about that. (Has anyone ever called you a "drama queen"?) *ALSO CONSIDER BEHAVIOR DURING INTERVIEW.* You've said that you are [*Are you*] more emotional than most other people, for example, sobbing when you hear a sad story. Tell me about that.

Commentary: People with this disorder tend to be very dramatic in telling stories about themselves or in expressing their emotions. They may embarrass friends and acquaintances by an excessive public display of emotions (e.g., embracing casual acquaintances with excessive ardor, sobbing uncontrollably on minor sentimental occasions, or having temper tantrums). This question can often be answered by observing the person's behavior during the assessment interview. Be careful not to include behavior that occurs only during Manic or Hypomanic Episodes.

7. Is suggestible (i.e., easily influenced by others or circumstances).

Interviewer's Questions: You've said that you [*Do you*] often change your mind about things depending on the people you're with or what you have just read or seen on TV. Tell me more about that.

Commentary: People with this characteristic tend to follow the latest fad, adopt new convictions easily, and quickly develop new "heroes." Their opinions and values are overly influenced by their peers, coworkers, family, and media. They appear to have no stable core of their own beliefs and values.

8. Considers relationships to be more intimate than they actually are.

> **Interviewer's Questions:** You've said that you *[Do you]* feel that you are good friends even with people who provide a service, like your plumber, your car mechanic, and your doctor. Tell me about that.

Commentary: This characteristic may be evident in the individual describing people as close friends even though he or she has just met them or had only a single conversation with them.

5.8 Narcissistic Personality Disorder

1. Has a grandiose sense of self-importance (e.g., exaggerates achievements and talents, expects to be recognized as superior without commensurate achievements).

> **Interviewer's Questions:** You've said that you are *[Are you]* more important, more talented, or more successful than most other people. Tell me about that. You've said that people have *[Have people]* told you that you have too high an opinion of yourself. Give me some examples of this.

Commentary: Individuals with Narcissistic Personality Disorder routinely overestimate their abilities and inflate their accomplishments, often appearing boastful and pretentious. They may blithely assume that others attribute the same value to their efforts and may be surprised when the praise they expect and feel they deserve is not forthcoming. Look for discrepancies between the person's expectation of recognition and his or her willingness to work or pass through ordinary hurdles (e.g., to get the required degree or go up through the ranks).

2. Is preoccupied with fantasies of unlimited success, power, brilliance, beauty, or ideal love.

> **Interviewer's Questions:** You've said that *[Do]* you think a lot about the power, success, or recognition that you expect to be yours someday. Tell me more about this. (How much time do you spend thinking about these things?) You've said that *[Do]* you think a lot about the perfect romance that will be yours someday. Tell me more about this. (How much time do you spend thinking about this?)

Commentary: In some people, this characteristic may be manifested by frequent daydreaming or other nonproductive activity that occurs in lieu of taking concrete steps toward reaching their aspirations of success, power, love, and so forth. For example, the person spends hours sitting around in a coffee shop talking about one day being a great novelist instead of spending the time writing. In others, there may be a preoccupation with activities that are ultimately fruitless because of the unachievable nature of the fantasies (e.g., a person who goes to singles bars every night looking for the perfect romance).

3. **Believes that he or she is "special" and unique and can only be understood by, or should associate with, other special or high-status people (or institutions).**

> **Interviewer's Questions:** You've said that when you have a problem, *[When you have a problem, do]* you almost always insist on seeing the top person. Give me some examples. (Why do you have to see the top person? Is it because you are unique or special? In what way?) You've said that *[Do]* you try to spend time with people who are important or influential. Why is that? (Is it because you are too special or unique to spend time with people who are not?)

Commentary: People with Narcissistic Personality Disorder consider themselves to be special, unique, and superior to others and will often limit their contacts to others whom they consider comparably special and talented. For example, a person with Narcissistic Personality Disorder may go to a party only after being assured that other "special" people will attend as well. As a consequence of their grandiose sense of self-importance and a sense that they deserve only the best, people with Narcissistic Personality Disorder often insist on seeing only the very top person (doctor, lawyer, hairdresser, teacher) or those from the most prestigious institutions.

4. **Requires excessive admiration.**

> **Interviewer's Questions:** You've said that it is *[Is it]* important to you that people pay attention to you or admire you in some way. Tell me more about this.

Commentary: The self-esteem of individuals with Narcissistic Personality Disorder is invariably very fragile and must be constantly bolstered by the attention and admiration of others. People with this disorder may report being preoccupied with concerns about how well they are doing and how others perceive them, or report feelings of dysphoria when they are not the object of attention or admiration.

5. **Has a sense of entitlement (i.e., unreasonable expectations of especially favorable treatment or automatic compliance with his or her expectations).**

> **Interviewer's Questions:** You've said that *[Do]* you feel that you are the kind of person who deserves special treatment or that other people should automatically do what you want. Tell me about that.

Commentary: It is important to make sure that the expectation of special treatment is truly unreasonable, taking into account the actual status of the person. Typically, the person feels entitled to special treatment because of his or her own intrinsic "specialness." For example, the person may assume that he or she does not have to wait in line because his needs are so important that others should defer to him.

6. **Is interpersonally exploitative (i.e., takes advantage of others to achieve his or her own ends).**

> **Interviewer's Questions:** You've said that *[Do]* you often have to put your needs above other people's. Give me some examples of when that happens. You've said

that others have *[Have others]* complained that you take advantage of people. Tell me about that.

Commentary: The combination of entitlement and lack of sensitivity to the needs of others often leads to the exploitation of others. People with Narcissistic Personality Disorder feel that they are so important and special that their needs deserve to be met no matter what the consequences are for others. For example, these individuals may expect great dedication from others and may overwork them without regard for the impact on their lives. They may establish friendships or romantic relationships with others only if these relationships are likely to enhance their self-esteem or further their goals.

7. **Lacks empathy: is unwilling to recognize or identify with the feelings and needs of others.**

   Interviewer's Questions: You've said that you *[Do you]* generally feel that other people's needs or feelings are really not your problem. Tell me about that. You've said that you *[Do you]* often find other people's problems to be boring. Tell me about that. You've said that people have *[Have people]* complained to you that you don't listen to them or care about their feelings. Tell me about that.

Commentary: People with Narcissistic Personality Disorder are generally oblivious to the concerns, needs, and welfare of others. They tend to dominate conversations, discussing their own concerns and interests in lengthy detail without regard for the feelings and needs of others. They are often contemptuous and impatient with others who talk about their own problems and concerns. These individuals may be oblivious to the hurt their remarks may inflict (e.g., exuberantly telling a former lover that "I am now in the relationship of a lifetime!"; boasting of health in front of someone who is sick). They may have the capacity to demonstrate empathy (e.g., a successful therapist with Narcissistic Personality Disorder) but do not demonstrate it unless it serves their own purposes.

8. **Is often envious of others or believes that others are envious of him or her.**

   Interviewer's Questions: You've said that when you see someone who is successful you *[When you see someone who is successful, do you]* feel that you deserve it more than they do. Give me some examples. (How often do you feel that way?) You've said that *[Do]* you feel that others are often envious of you. What do they envy about you?

Commentary: People with Narcissistic Personality Disorder are constantly judging how well they measure up to others. They often devalue, begrudge, or denigrate others' successes, feeling that they better deserve the admiration or privileges. They may harshly devalue the contributions of others, particularly when those individuals have received acknowledgment or praise for their accomplishments. In some cases, they may assume that others must be envious of them.

9. **Shows arrogant, haughty behaviors or attitudes.**

> **Interviewer's Questions:** You've said that you [*Do you*] find that there are very few people who are worth your time and attention. Tell me about that. *ALSO CONSIDER BEHAVIOR DURING INTERVIEW* You've said that other people have complained [*Have other people complained*] that you act too "high and mighty" or arrogant. Tell me about that.

Commentary: The interviewer should look for evidence of snobbish or patronizing attitudes or behaviors. These attitudes are often evident during the interview; for example, the person makes disdainful comments about the interviewer's style, appearance, or the interview itself (e.g., "Who thought up these stupid questions?").

5.9   Borderline Personality Disorder

1. **Frantic efforts to avoid real or imagined abandonment. (Note: Do not include suicidal or self-mutilating behavior covered in Criterion 5.)**

> **Interviewer's Questions:** You've said that you have [*Have you*] become frantic when you thought that someone you really cared about was going to leave you. What have you done? (Have you threatened or pleaded with him/her?) How often has this happened?

Commentary: In individuals with Borderline Personality Disorder, the perception of impending separation or rejection, or the loss of external structure, can lead to profound changes in self-image, affect, cognition, and behavior. This criterion specifically refers to frantic actions taken by the person in order to keep someone that they are involved with, attached to, or dependent on from leaving. Examples of such behavior include pleading with someone not to leave or physically restraining the person who is attempting to leave. As indicated in the note, suicidal or self-mutilating behavior that occurs in response to threats of abandonment is already covered by Criterion 5. If such behavior is the only manifestation of the person's efforts to avoid abandonment, this criterion should be rated "0." Note that individuals with Dependent Personality Disorder may also become frantic if the person on whom they depend for support or nurturance is going to leave them. If the efforts to avoid real or threatened abandonment are driven entirely by these concerns, this criterion should not be rated "2."

2. **A pattern of unstable and intense interpersonal relationships characterized by alternating between extremes of idealization and devaluation.**

> **Interviewer's Questions:** You've said that [*Do*] relationships with people you really care about have lots of extreme ups and downs. Tell me about them. (Were there times when you thought these people were perfect or everything you wanted, and then other times when you thought they were terrible? How many relationships have been like this?)

Commentary: There are three necessary components to this criterion. First, there must be a pattern of unstable relationships, characterized by frequent conflict and threats of separation (or actual periods of separation). Second, these relationships must be intense, in that strong emotions must be present (such as euphoria, infatuation, anger, resentment, despair). Finally, the person must relate to the other person in the relationship with overidealization at times and devaluation at other times. For example, a person with Borderline Personality Disorder may idealize potential caregivers or lovers at the first or second meeting, demand to spend a lot of time together, and share the most intimate details early in a relationship. However, that person will then switch quickly from idealizing the other person to devaluing them, feeling that the other person does not care enough, does not give enough, or is not "there" enough. In analytic terms, these individuals commonly use splitting as a defense mechanism.

3. **Identity disturbance: markedly and persistently unstable self-image or sense of self.**

   Interviewer's Questions: You've said that your sense of who you are often changes *[Does your sense of who you are often change]* dramatically. Tell me more about that. You've said that you are *[Are you]* different with different people or in different situations, so that you sometimes don't know who you really are. Give me some examples of this. (Do you feel this way a lot?) You've said that there have been *[Have there been]* lots of sudden changes in your goals, career plans, religious beliefs, and so on. Tell me more about that. You've said that there have been *[Have there been]* lots of sudden changes in the kinds of friends you have or in your sexual identity. Tell me more about that.

   Commentary: Identity is a stable sense of self providing a unity of personality over time. The type of identity disturbance that is characteristic of Borderline Personality Disorder consists of extreme shifts in the person's sense of who he or she is, which is often manifested in abrupt changes in jobs or career goals, reported sexual orientation, personal values, friends, or the person's fundamental sense of self (e.g., as evil or good). Note that this criterion should be rated "2" only if the identity disturbance is not appropriate for the person's developmental age (i.e., normal adolescent identity shifts should not be considered).

4. **Impulsivity in at least two areas that are potentially self-damaging (e.g., spending, sex, substance abuse, reckless driving, binge eating). (Note: Do not include suicidal or self-mutilating behavior covered in Criterion 5.)**

   Interviewer's Questions: You've said that you've *[Have you]* often done things impulsively. What kinds of things? (How about…buying things you really couldn't afford?…having sex with people you hardly knew or having "unsafe sex"?…drinking too much or taking drugs?…driving recklessly?…uncontrollable eating?) *IF YES TO ANY OF ABOVE:* Tell me about that. How often does it happen?

Commentary: The central feature of this criterion is the person's inability to exercise control over his or her impulses to engage in behavior that is gratifying in the short run but potentially destructive in the long run. Note that the behaviors listed in the questions are merely examples and are not intended to be exhaustive. In this list, "spending" refers to the impulsive buying of things the person cannot really afford, and "sex" refers to impulsively deciding to have sex with someone (or having "unsafe sex") without considering potentially self-damaging consequences. Per the note that appears with this criterion, impulsive suicidal or self-mutilating behavior does not count toward meeting the requirement of "two areas that are potentiality self-damaging" because such behavior is covered in Criterion 5.

5. **Recurrent suicidal behavior, gestures, or threats, or self-mutilating behavior.**

   Interviewer's Questions: You've said that you have *[Have you]* tried to hurt or kill yourself or threatened to do so. *IF YES:* When was the last time that happened? You've said that you have *[Have you ever]* cut, burned, or scratched yourself on purpose. Tell me about that.

   Commentary: Do not rate this criterion "2" for a person who simply tells others about passive suicidal ideation ("I wish I were dead"). "Self-mutilating behavior" refers to physically self-injurious behavior without any suicidal intent. Common examples include wrist-cutting, scratching, or burning himself or herself with a cigarette. These self-destructive acts are usually precipitated by threats of separation or rejection or by expectations that the individual assume increased responsibility. Self-mutilation may occur during dissociative experiences and often brings relief by reaffirming the ability to feel or by expiating the individual's sense of being evil.

6. **Affective instability due to a marked reactivity of mood (e.g., intense episodic dysphoria, irritability, or anxiety usually lasting a few hours and only rarely more than a few days).**

   Interviewer's Questions: You've said that your mood often changes *[Does your mood often change]* in a single day, based on what's going on in your life. Tell me about that. What kinds of things cause your mood to change? How long do your "bad" moods typically last?

   Commentary: Affective instability refers to the shifting, unstable quality of the person's mood. The basic dysphoric mood of those with Borderline Personality Disorder is often disrupted by periods of anger, panic, or despair and is rarely relieved by periods of well-being or satisfaction. Although the change in mood is often abrupt, a sudden onset of the mood change is not a requirement. Instead, this criterion specifies frequent mood changes that are of a large magnitude but of a relatively brief duration—hours, rather than days or weeks.

7. Chronic feelings of emptiness.

> **Interviewer's Questions:** You've said that *[Do]* you often feel empty inside. Tell me more about this.

Commentary: The chronic feelings of emptiness are often associated with feelings of being bored, hollow, alone, or without definition.

8. Inappropriate, intense anger or difficulty controlling anger (e.g., frequent displays of temper, constant anger, recurrent physical fights).

> **Interviewer's Questions:** You've said that *[Do]* you often have temper outbursts or get so angry that you lose control. Give me some examples. You've said that *[Do]* you hit people or throw things when you get angry. Give me some examples. (Does this happen often?) You've said that *[Do]* even little things get you very angry. Give me some examples. (Does this happen often?)

Commentary: "Inappropriate anger" refers to the intensity of the person's anger being out of proportion to the cause. Lack of control of anger may be evidenced by extreme physical displays such as hitting people or throwing things. The anger often is expressed in the context of real or perceived lack of caring, deprivation, or abandonment.

9. Transient, stress-related paranoid ideation or severe dissociative symptoms.

> **Interviewer's Questions:** You've said that when you get very upset, you *[When you get very upset, do you]* get suspicious of other people or feel disconnected from your body or that things are unreal. In what kinds of situations has this happened?

Commentary: During periods of stress, some people with Borderline Personality Disorder develop transient paranoid or dissociative symptoms that are rarely severe enough to warrant an additional diagnosis (e.g., Brief Psychotic Disorder). In cases in which paranoid ideation is persistent and not related to periods of stress, a diagnosis of Paranoid Personality Disorder should be considered instead. The stressor is often real, perceived, or anticipated withdrawal of care or attention of a caregiver (e.g., lover, parent, therapist). In such situations, the real or perceived return of the caregiver's nurturance may result in a remission of the symptoms. The dissociative symptoms include periods of dissociative amnesia (sometimes manifested by the person having the feeling that he or she has lost time), depersonalization (i.e., a feeling of detachment or estrangement from one's self), or derealization (i.e., the sense that the external world is unreal or strange). These episodes typically last minutes or hours.

5.10 Antisocial Personality Disorder

C. There is evidence of Conduct Disorder with onset before age 15 years.

The DSM-5 text (p. 659) explicating Criterion C for Antisocial Personality Disorder indicates that there must have been "some symptoms of Conduct Disorder before age 15" without indicating how many Conduct Disorder criteria are required. The SCID-5-PD has operationalized Criterion C to require at least two symptoms of Conduct Disorder on the basis of the following rationale: the use of "some symptoms" in the DSM-5 text implies that more than one symptom is required, whereas a requirement of three symptoms would be at the DSM-5 diagnostic threshold for Conduct Disorder. The following items 1–15 assessed in Criterion C for Antisocial Personality Disorder in the SCID-5-PD reflect DSM-5 Criteria A1–A15 for Conduct Disorder.

1. **[Before the age of 15] often bullied, threatened, or intimidated others.**

   Interviewer's Questions: You've said that before you were 15, you bullied, threatened, or scared [*Before you were 15, did you bully, threaten, or scare*] other kids. Give me some examples. How often did this happen?

   Commentary: The implied threat must be of physical harm and not simply withdrawal of friendship.

2. **[Before the age of 15] often initiated physical fights.**

   Interviewer's Questions: You've said that before you were 15, you started [*Before you were 15, did you start*] fights. Give me some examples. How often did this happen?

   Commentary: This criterion should be rated "2" only if there is evidence that the person started fights, rather than just being drawn into them.

3. **[Before the age of 15] has used a weapon that can cause serious physical harm to others (e.g., a bat, brick, broken bottle, knife, gun).**

   Interviewer's Questions: You've said that before you were 15, you hurt or threatened someone [*Before you were 15, did you hurt or threaten someone*] with a weapon, like a bat, brick, broken bottle, a knife or a gun. Tell me about that.

   Commentary: Any use of a weapon that has the potential to cause serious physical harm warrants a rating of "2" and ranges from using a weapon in a fight to using a weapon to threaten, intimidate, rob, or sexually assault someone.

4. **[Before the age of 15] has been physically cruel to people.**

   Interviewer's Questions: You've said that before you were 15, you did [*Before you were 15, did you do*] cruel things to someone that caused him or her physical pain or suffering. What did you do?

Commentary: This criterion refers to torturing or inflicting pain and suffering on others apart from injuries inflicted during a fight. It may also include situations in which no actual physical pain is inflicted (e.g., locking a child in a closet).

5. **[Before the age of 15] has been physically cruel to animals.**

   Interviewer's Questions: You've said that before you were 15, *[Before you were 15, did]* you hurt animals on purpose. What did you do?

   Commentary: Being "physically cruel" implies purposely inflicting pain and suffering on the animal.

6. **[Before the age of 15] has stolen while confronting a victim (e.g., mugging, purse snatching, extortion, armed robbery).**

   Interviewer's Questions: You've said that before you were 15, you robbed, mugged, or took *[Before you were 15, did you mug, rob, or forcibly take]* something from someone by threatening him or her. Tell me about that.

   Commentary: This criterion requires face-to-face confrontation ranging from verbal threats to actual violence.

7. **[Before the age of 15] has forced someone into sexual activity.**

   Interviewer's Questions: You've said that before you were 15, you forced *[Before you were 15, did you force]* someone to do something sexual. Tell me about that.

   Commentary: This criterion refers to any coerced sexual activity ranging from forcing someone to watch a sexual act, forcing someone to undress, forcing someone to touch the subject sexually, to forcing someone into sexual intercourse without that person's consent (rape).

8. **[Before the age of 15] has deliberately engaged in fire setting with the intention of causing serious damage.**

   Interviewer's Questions: You've said that before you were 15, *[Before you were 15, did]* you set fires. Tell me about that. Were you hoping to cause serious damage?

   Commentary: What is critical is the intention, rather than whether or not the fire actually caused severe damage.

9. **[Before the age of 15] has deliberately destroyed others' property (other than by fire setting).**

   Interviewer's Questions: You've said that before you were 15, you deliberately destroyed *[Before you were 15, did you deliberately destroy]* things that weren't yours. What did you do?

Commentary: This criterion refers to vandalism of property with the intent to destroy, rather than purely as a form of expression (i.e., graffiti-writing on a wall would not count, but breaking windows, trashing a house, putting dirt in a gas tank, or slashing tires would count). Fire setting is excluded from this criterion because it is covered in the previous criterion.

10. [Before the age of 15] has broken into someone else's house, building, or car.

Interviewer's Questions: You've said that before you were 15, you broke *[Before you were 15, did you break]* into houses, other buildings, or cars. Tell me about that.

11. [Before the age of 15] often lies to obtain goods or favors or to avoid obligations (i.e., "cons" others).

Interviewer's Questions: You've said that before you were 15, you lied a lot or conned *[Before you were 15, did you lie a lot or con]* other people to get something you wanted or to get out of doing something. Give me some examples. How often did you do that?

Commentary: This criterion refers to manipulative lying. What is not included is lying for other reasons, such as to avoid harsh punishment, to get someone else in trouble, or to keep one's parents at a distance.

12. [Before the age of 15] has stolen items of nontrivial value without confronting a victim (e.g., shoplifting, [stealing] but without breaking and entering; forgery).

Interviewer's Questions: You've said that before you were 15, you sometimes shoplifted, stole something, or forged *[Before you were 15, did you sometimes shoplift, steal something, or forge]* someone's signature for money. Give me some examples.

Commentary: Not included is stealing of trivial items (e.g., candy) or forging a signature for purposes other than theft.

13. [Before the age of 15] has run away from home overnight at least twice while living in the parental or parental surrogate home, or once without returning for a lengthy period.

Interviewer's Questions: You've said that before you were 15, you ran away from home and stayed *[Before you were 15, did you run away and stay]* away overnight. Was that more than once? (With whom were you living at the time?)

Commentary: Note that runaway episodes that occur as a direct consequence of physical or sexual abuse would not qualify for a rating of "2."

14. [Before the age of 13] often stayed out at night despite parental prohibitions.

Interviewer's Questions: You've said that before you were 13, you would *[Before you were 13, did you]* often stay out very late, long after the time you were supposed to be home. How often?

15. [Before the age of 13] was often truant from school.

> **Interviewer's Questions:** You've said that before you were 13, you often skipped [*Before you were 13, did you often skip*] school. How often?

A. A pervasive pattern of disregard for and violation of the rights of others, occurring since age 15 years, as indicated by three (or more) of the following:

A1. Failure to conform to social norms with respect to lawful behaviors, as indicated by repeatedly performing acts that are grounds for arrest.

> **Interviewer's Questions:** Have you done things that are against the law—even if you weren't caught—like stealing, identity theft, writing bad checks, or having sex for money? *IF NOT KNOWN FROM OVERVIEW:* Have you ever been arrested for anything?

Commentary: Individuals with Antisocial Personality Disorder may repeatedly perform acts that are grounds for arrest (whether they are arrested or not), such as destroying property, harassing others, stealing, or pursuing illegal occupations. Note that this criterion refers to the social norms of the society at large (as defined by existing laws) as opposed to a subgroup that may condone certain illegal behavior. The acts, however, must be antisocial in nature; not included are acts of civil disobedience (e.g., trespassing while protesting).

A2. Deceitfulness, as indicated by repeated lying, use of aliases, or conning others for personal profit or pleasure.

> **Interviewer's Questions:** Do you often lie to get what you want or just for the fun of it? Have you ever used an alias or pretended you were someone else? Have you "conned" others to get something?

Commentary: Individuals with this trait have no regard for the truth and lie in order to exploit others or to maintain control over them. They are frequently deceitful and manipulative in order to gain personal profit or pleasure (e.g., to obtain money, sex, or power). This criterion does not include lying to protect the person from harm (e.g., from spousal abuse).

A3. Impulsivity or failure to plan ahead.

> **Interviewer's Questions:** Do you often do something on the spur of the moment without thinking about how it will affect you or other people? Tell me about that. What kinds of things? Did you ever walk off a job without having another one to go to? (How many times?) Have you ever moved out of a place without having another place to live? (Tell me about that.)

Commentary: This trait involves making decisions on the spur of the moment, without forethought and without consideration for the consequences to self or others; this may lead to sudden changes of jobs, residences, or relationships. Note that a rating of "2" requires that the lack of planning be clearly irresponsible and not merely evidence of spontaneity.

A4. Irritability and aggressiveness, as indicated by repeated physical fights or assaults.

> **Interviewer's Questions:** Have you been in any fights? (How often?) Have you ever been so angry that you hit or threw things at other people (INCLUDING SPOUSE/ PARTNER)? (How many times?) Have you ever hit a child very hard? Tell me about that. Have you physically threatened or hurt anyone else? Tell me about that. (How often?)

Commentary: Individuals with Antisocial Personality Disorder tend to be irritable and aggressive and may repeatedly get into physical fights or commit acts of physical assault (including beating a spouse or child). Aggressive acts that are required to defend oneself or someone else or that are required by the person's job are not included as evidence for this criterion.

A5. Reckless disregard for safety of self or others.

> **Interviewer's Questions:** Did you ever drive a car when you were drunk or high? How many speeding tickets have you gotten or car accidents have you been in? Do you always use protection if you have sex with someone you don't know well? (Has anyone ever said that you allowed a child to be in danger when you were supposed to be taking care of the child?)

Commentary: Individuals with Antisocial Personality Disorder display a reckless disregard for the safety of themselves or others. This may be evidenced in their driving behavior (e.g., recurrent speeding, driving while intoxicated, multiple accidents). They may engage in sexual behavior or substance use that has a high risk for harmful consequences. They may neglect or fail to care for a child in a way that puts the child in danger (e.g., allowing a child to wander onto a highway).

A6. Consistent irresponsibility, as indicated by repeated failure to sustain consistent work behavior or honor financial obligations.

> **Interviewer's Questions:** How much of the time in the last 5 years were you not working? *IF FOR A PROLONGED PERIOD:* Why? (Was there work available?) When you were working, did you miss a lot of work? *IF YES:* Why? Have you ever owed people money and not paid them back? (How often?) What about not paying child support or not giving money to children or someone else who depended on you?

Commentary: There must be evidence of either irresponsible work behavior or financial irresponsibility. Irresponsible work behavior may be indicated by significant periods of unemployment despite available job opportunities, abandonment of several jobs without a realistic plan for getting another job, or repeated absences from work not explained by illness. Financial irresponsibility may be indicated by repeatedly defaulting on debts, refusing to pay child support or alimony, or repeated squandering of money required for household food or other necessities.

A7. Lack of remorse, as indicated by being indifferent to or rationalizing having hurt, mistreated, or stolen from another.

> **Interviewer's Questions:** *IF THERE IS EVIDENCE OF ANTISOCIAL ACTS AND IT IS UNCLEAR WHETHER THERE IS ANY REMORSE:* How do you feel about (AN-TISOCIAL ACTS)? (Do you think what you did was wrong in any way?) Do you think you were justified in (ANTISOCIAL ACTS)? (Do you think the other person deserved it?)

Commentary: Individuals with Antisocial Personality Disorder show little remorse for the consequences of their acts. They may be indifferent to, or provide a superficial rationalization for, having hurt, mistreated, or stolen from someone (e.g., "life's unfair," "losers deserve to lose"). These individuals may blame the victims for being foolish, helpless, or deserving of their fate (e.g., "he had it coming anyway"); they may minimize the harmful consequences of their actions; or they may simply indicate complete indifference. They may believe that everyone is out to "help Number One" and that they should stop at nothing to avoid being pushed around.

6. Training

Ideally, training should involve the following sequence:

1. Study the *User's Guide for the SCID-5-PD,* familiarizing yourself with the basic features and conventions.
2. Carefully read through every word of the SCID-5-PD, making sure that you understand all of the instructions, the questions, and the diagnostic criteria. As you are reading through each criterion, refer to the corresponding item-by-item commentary.
3. Now practice reading the SCID-5-PD questions aloud so that eventually it sounds as if SCID-5-PD is your mother tongue.
4. Watch the example videos for the SCID-5-PD, making your own ratings as you go along. Then compare your ratings with the reference ratings provided with the video. Videos can be ordered on the SCID Web site (www.scid5.org).
5. Try out the SCID-5-PD with a colleague (or significant other) who can assume the role of a subject.
6. Try out the SCID-5-PD on actual subjects who are as representative as possible of those who will be included in your research study. If possible, these rehearsals should be joint interviews with all raters making independent ratings, followed by a discussion of the interviewing technique and all sources of disagreement in the ratings.
7. If possible, do a test-retest reliability study in which the interview is repeated with the same subject within a short period of time by a second independent interviewer. You will learn more from such a study if you audiotape the interviews, then have

each interviewer listen to and rate the audiotape of the other interviewer, followed by a discussion of sources of disagreement.

A test-retest reliability study may be impractical for some investigators. A less rigorous procedure for assessing the reliability of interviewers is to make a series of audio- or videotapes. In general, we would recommend a minimum of 10 joint interviews, although the more the better.

8. Investigators who are planning studies may wish to contact the SCID-5-PD authors (scid5@columbia.edu) about conducting a training workshop at your site (which would focus on direct supervision of live interviews) or reviewing a series of taped interviews made by your interviewers.

7. Reliability and Validity

7.1 Reliability of the SCID-5-PD

At the time of publication of this *User's Guide,* no data were available on the reliability or validity of the SCID-5-PD. A number of studies, however, have investigated the reliability of its predecessors, the SCID-II for DSM-III-R and the SCID-II for DSM-IV (see Table 7–1). Reliability for categorical constructs, such as the DSM diagnoses assessed in the SCID-5-PD, is reported in terms of kappa, a statistic that corrects for chance agreement. Kappa values above 0.70 are considered to indicate good agreement; values from 0.50 to 0.70, fair agreement; and below 0.50, poor agreement. In addition to determining diagnostic agreement at a categorical level, several studies (e.g., Dreessen and Arntz 1998; Lobbestael et al. 2011; Weertman et al. 2003) also determined diagnostic agreement of the dimensionalized versions of the DSM Personality Disorders, which is measured using the intraclass correlation coefficient (ICC). Note that these studies dimensionalized the Personality Disorders both as a sum of the number of items scored positively, referred to as the "trait ICC" in Table 7–1, and the total score of the ratings for the disorder (i.e., including both threshold and subthreshold ratings, as is done in the SCID-5-PD), referred to as the "sum ICC" in Table 7–1. Note that in order for the kappa statistic to be calculated, the base rate must be above a minimum threshold because diagnostic disagreements have an inordinately pronounced effect on reliability when the base rate is either too high or too low. In such cases, kappa values were not reported (and are indicated by "***" in Table 7–1).

As can be seen in Table 7–1, the range of kappas from different studies and for different diagnoses is quite large. Many factors influence the reliability of an interview instrument such as the SCID-5-PD. We will address some of these below.

Joint Interviews or Test-Retest Design

In some studies, a subject is interviewed by one clinician, while others observe (either in person or by reviewing a tape) and then make independent ratings. Joint interviews produce the highest reliability because all raters are hearing exactly the same story and observing the same interview behaviors, and because the adherence to skip instructions provides clues to the observers regarding the ratings made by the interviewer. A

TABLE 7–1. Summary of selected SCID-II reliability studies

Study	First et al. 1995	Weiss et al. 1995	Arntz et al. 1992	Dreessen and Arntz 1998	Maffei et al. 1997	Osone and Takahashi 2003	Weertman et. al. 2003	Lobbestael et al. 2011
N	284	31	70	43	231	120	69	151
Method	1–3 week interval, test-retest	12-month interval, test-retest	Joint with live observer	1–4 week interval, test-retest	Joint with live observer	12-month interval, test-retest	1–6 week interval, test-retest	Joint with audiotape
Statistic	kappa	kappa	kappa	kappa/trait ICC/sum ICC	kappa	kappa	kappa/trait ICC/sum ICC	kappa/trait ICC/sum ICC
Version	DSM-III-R (U.S.)	DSM-III-R (U.S.)	DSM-III-R (Dutch)	DSM-III-R (Dutch)	DSM-IV (Italian)	DSM-IV (Japanese)	DSM-IV (Dutch)	DSM-IV (Dutch)
Type of Personality Disorder								
Avoidant	0.54	–0.15	0.82	0.73/0.80/0.80	0.97	0.93	0.79/0.82/0.82	0.83/0.89/0.90
Dependent	0.50	0.43	1	***/0.49/0.64	0.86	0.66	***/0.20/0.38	0.83/0.90/0.92
Obsessive-Compulsive	0.24	0.26	0.72	***/0.75/0.84	0.83	0.86	***/0.63/0.62	0.87/0.87/0.89
Passive-Aggressive/ Negativistic	0.47	0.71	0.66	***/0.62/0.60	0.91	***	***	***/0.85/0.86
Self-Defeating	0.33	***	1	***/0.53/0.53	**	**	**	**
Depressive	*	*	*	*				
Paranoid	0.57	0.47	0.77	***/0.66/0.63	0.93	0.74	***/0.71/0.76	0.94/0.94/0.95
Schizotypal	0.54	0.78	0.65	***/0.59/0.71	0.91	0.49	***	***/0.85/0.85
Schizoid	***	***	***	***/***/***	0.91	1.0	***	***/0.62/0.69
Histrionic	0.62	0.59	0.85	***/0.24/0.36	0.92	0.80	***	***/0.76/0.78
Narcissistic	0.42	0.59	1	***/***/***	0.98	0.74	***	***/0.75/0.72
Borderline	0.48	0.02	0.79	***/0.72/0.75	0.91	0.85	***/0.70/0.71	0.91/0.93/0.95
Antisocial	0.76	0.41	***	***/0.75/0.70	0.95	0.89	***/0.88/0.87	0.78/0.78/0.85

Note. ICC=intraclass correlation coefficient; SCID-II=Structured Clinical Interview for DSM Axis II Personality Disorders.
* Not included in SCID-II for DSM-III-R (Spitzer et al. 1990).
** Not included in SCID-II for DSM-IV (First et al. 1997).
*** Not reported because too few cases.

more stringent test of reliability, a test-retest design entails having the same subject interviewed at two different times by two different interviewers (or at two different points in time by the same rater). The test-retest method tends to lead to lower levels of reliability because the subject may, even when prompted by the same questions, tell different stories to the two interviewers (information variance), resulting in divergent ratings.

Interviewer Training

Raters who are well trained, and particularly raters who train and work together, are likely to have better agreement on ratings. It is worth noting that the professional discipline of the interviewer (e.g., psychiatrist, psychologist, social worker) does not appear to contribute to differences in reliability.

Subject Population

Subjects with more severe Personality Disorders (such as patients hospitalized for their Personality Disorder) are likely to yield more reliable SCID-5-PD diagnoses than subjects with milder Personality Disorders that border on normality. This reflects the fact that relatively minor diagnostic disagreements are more likely to have a profound effect on the diagnosis when the severity of the disorder is just at the diagnostic threshold. For example, a disagreement about a single criterion for a subject meeting exactly five out of nine criteria of Borderline Personality Disorder makes the difference between a diagnosis of Borderline Personality Disorder or of Other Specified Personality Disorder, whereas a one-criterion disagreement for a patient meeting seven out of nine criteria would not result in any apparent disagreement on the diagnosis.

Base Rates

The base rates of the diagnoses in the population being studied affect the reported reliability. If the error of measurement for a diagnostic instrument is constant, reliability varies directly with the base rates. It is thus harder to obtain good reliability for a rare diagnosis than for a common diagnosis.

7.2   Validity of the SCID-II

Skodol and colleagues (1988) compared results of a personality assessment using the SCID-II with a LEAD standard (Spitzer 1983). The LEAD standard involves conducting a longitudinal assessment (L) (i.e., relying on data collected over time), done by expert diagnosticians (E), using all data (AD) that are available about the subject, such as family informants, review of medical records, and observations of clinical staff. Skodol et al. (1988) found that the diagnostic power (ratio of true test results to total number of tests administered) of the SCID-II (Spitzer et al. 1990) varies by diagnosis (from 0.45 for Narcissistic Personality Disorder to 0.95 for Antisocial Personality Disorder), with the diagnostic power being 0.85 or greater for five Personality Disorders. Several studies (O'Boyle and Self 1990; Oldham et al. 1992; Renneberg et al. 1992) comparing the

SCID-II with other measures of personality (e.g., Millon Clinical Multiaxial Inventory, Personality Disorder Examination) have shown rather poor agreement between the instruments, although no conclusion could be reached about which instrument was more valid. Ryder and colleagues (2007) used the SCID-II to evaluate DSM-IV Personality Disorder items with respect to convergent validity, divergent validity, relation to general personality traits, and association with functional impairment. They found that only Borderline Personality Disorder items were satisfactory on all four evaluation criteria. It should be noted that this study was designed to look at the validity of the DSM-IV Personality Disorders, rather than the SCID-II instrument itself.

7.3 Psychometric Properties of the SCID-II Patient Questionnaire

Three studies (Ekselius et al. 1994; Jacobsberg et al. 1995; Nussbaum and Rogers 1992) examined the sensitivity and specificity of the SCID-II-PQ when used as a screening tool, confirming a very low rate of false negatives. Although the SCID-II-PQ was not designed as a stand-alone instrument, Ekselius and colleagues (1994) were able to determine cutoff scores for the SCID-II-PQ that resulted in Personality Disorder diagnoses that were similar to those obtained by the SCID-II interview, with an overall kappa of agreement of 0.78. Ball and colleagues (2001), also using the SCID-II-PQ as a stand-alone instrument, found the mean internal consistency of SCID-II-PQ-rated Personality Disorders in a population to be above 0.6 (the lowest acceptable value), with internal consistencies ranging from 0.35 to 0.80, and acceptable values for all disorders except for Schizoid, Schizotypal, Histrionic, and Obsessive-Compulsive Personality Disorders.

References

American Psychiatric Association: Diagnostic and Statistical Manual of Mental Disorders, 3rd Edition (DSM-III). Washington, DC, American Psychiatric Association, 1994

American Psychiatric Association: Diagnostic and Statistical Manual of Mental Disorders, 3rd Edition, Revised (DSM-III-R). Washington, DC, American Psychiatric Association, 1994

American Psychiatric Association: Diagnostic and Statistical Manual of Mental Disorders, 4th Edition (DSM-IV). Washington, DC, American Psychiatric Association, 1994

American Psychiatric Association: Diagnostic and Statistical Manual of Mental Disorders, 4th Edition, Text Revision (DSM-IV-TR). Washington, DC, American Psychiatric Association, 1994

American Psychiatric Association: Diagnostic and Statistical Manual of Mental Disorders, 5th Edition (DSM-5). Arlington, VA, American Psychiatric Association, 2013

Arntz A, van Beijsterveldt B, Hoekstra R, Hofman A, et al: The interrater reliability of a Dutch version of the Structured Clinical Interview for DSM-III-R Personality Disorders. Acta Psychiatr Scand 85(5):394–400, 1992

Ball SA, Rounsaville BJ, Tennen H, Kranzler HR: Reliability of personality disorder symptoms and personality traits in substance-dependent inpatients. J Abnorm Psychol 110(2):341–352, 2001

Calderone A, Mauri M, Calabrò PF, Piaggi P, et al: Exploring the concept of eating dyscontrol in severely obese patients candidate to bariatric surgery. Clin Obes 5(1):22–30, 2015

Casadio P, Olivoni D, Ferrari B, Pintori C, et al: Personality disorders in addiction outpatients: prevalence and effects on psychosocial functioning. Subst Abuse 8:17–24, 2014

Dreessen L, Arntz A. Short-interval test-retest interrater reliability of the Structured Clinical Interview for DSM-III-R personality disorders (SCID-II) in outpatients. J Pers Disord 12(2):138–148, 1998

Edens JF, Kelley SE, Lilienfeld SO, Skeem JL, et al: DSM-5 antisocial personality disorder: predictive validity in a prison sample. Law Hum Behav 39(2):123–129, 2015

Ekselius L, Lindstrom E, von Knorring L, Bodlund O, et al: SCID II interviews and the SCID Screen questionnaire as diagnostic tools for personality disorders in DSM-III-R. Acta Psychiatr Scand 90(2):120–123, 1994

First MB, Spitzer RL, Gibbon M, Williams JBW, et al: The Structured Clinical Interview for DSM-III-R Personality Disorders (SCID-II). Part II: multi-site test-retest reliability study. J Pers Disord 9(2):92–104, 1995

First MB, Gibbon M, Spitzer RL, Williams JBW, et al: Structured Clinical Interview for DSM-IV Axis II Personality Disorders (SCID-II). Washington, DC, American Psychiatric Press, 1997

Gremaud-Heitz D, Riemenschneider A, Walter M, Sollberger D, et al: Comorbid atypical depression in borderline personality disorder is common and correlated with anxiety-related psychopathology. Compr Psychiatry 55(3):650–656, 2014

Huprich SK, Paggeot AV, Samuel DB: Comparing the Personality Disorder Interview for DSM-IV (PDI-IV) and SCID-II borderline personality disorder scales: an item-response theory analysis. J Pers Assess 97(1):13–21, 2015

Jacobsberg L, Perry S, Frances A: Diagnostic agreement between the SCID-II screening questionnaire and the Personality Disorder Examination. J Pers Assess 65(3):428–433, 1995

Lobbestael J, Leurgans M, Arntz A: Inter-rater reliability of the Structured Clinical Interview for DSM-IV Axis I Disorders (SCID I) and Axis II Disorders (SCID II). Clin Psychol Psychother 18(1):75–79, 2011

Maffei C, Fossati A, Agostoni I, Barraco A, et al: Interrater reliability and internal consistency of the Structured Clinical Interview for DSM-IV Axis II personality disorders (SCID-II), version 2.0. J Pers Disord 11(3):279–284, 1997

Martín-Blanco A, Ferrer M, Soler J, Salazar J, et al: Association between methylation of the glucocorticoid receptor gene, childhood maltreatment, and clinical severity in borderline personality disorder. J Psychiatr Res 57:34–40, 2014

Mulder RT, Joyce PR, Frampton CM: Personality disorders improve in patients treated for major depression. Acta Psychiatr Scand 122(3):219–225, 2010

Nussbaum D, Rogers R: Screening psychiatric patients for Axis II disorders. Can J Psychiatry 37:658–660, 1992

O'Boyle M, Self D: Comparison of two interviews for DSM-III-R personality disorders. Psychiatry Res 32:85–92, 1990

Odlaug BL, Schreiber LR, Grant JE: Personality disorders and dimensions in pathological gambling. J Pers Disord 26(3):381–392, 2012

Oldham JM, Skodol AE: Charting the future of Axis II. J Pers Disord 14:17–29, 2000

Oldham JM, Skodol AE, Kellman HD, Hyler SE, et al: Diagnosis of DSM-III-R personality disorders by two structured interviews: patterns of comorbidity. Am J Psychiatry 149(2):213–220, 1992

Osone A, Takahashi S: Twelve month test-retest reliability of a Japanese version of the Structured Clinical Interview for DSM-IV Personality Disorders. Psychiatry Clin Neurosciences 57(5):532–538, 2003

Renneberg B, Chambless DL, Dowdall DJ, Fauerbach JA, et al: A structured interview for DSM-III-R, Axis II, and the Millon Clinical Multiaxial Inventory: a concurrent validity study of personality disorders among anxious outpatients. J Pers Disord 6(2):117–124, 1992

Rojas EC, Cummings JR, Bornovalova MA, Hopwood CJ, et al: A further validation of the Minnesota Borderline Personality Disorder Scale. Personal Disord 5(2):146–153, 2014

Ryder AG, Costa PT, Bagby RM: Evaluation of the SCID-II personality disorder traits for DSM-IV: coherence, discrimination, relations with general personality traits, and functional impairment. J Pers Disord 21(6):626–637, 2007

Sharp C, Wright AG, Fowler JC, Frueh BC, et al: The structure of personality pathology: both general ('g') and specific ('s') factors? J Abnorm Psychol 124(2):387–398, 2015

Skodol AE, Rosnick L, Kellman D, Oldham JM, et al: Validating structured DSM-III-R personality disorder assessments with longitudinal data. Am J Psychiatry 145:1297–1299, 1988

Spitzer RL: Psychiatric diagnosis: are clinicians still necessary? Compr Psychiatry 24(5):399–411, 1983

Spitzer RL, Williams JBW, Gibbon M, First MB: Structured Clinical Interview for DSM-III-R Axis II Disorders (SCID-II). Washington, DC, American Psychiatric Press, 1990

Uguz F, Engin B, Yilmaz E: Quality of life in patients with chronic idiopathic urticaria: the impact of Axis I and Axis II psychiatric disorders. Gen Hosp Psychiatry 30(5):453–457, 2008

Weertman A, Arntz A, Dreessen L, van Velzen C, et al: Short-interval test-retest interrater reliability of the Dutch version of the Structured Clinical Interview for DSM-IV personality disorders (SCID-II). J Pers Disord 17(6):562–567, 2003

Weiss RD, Najavits LM, Muenz LR, Hufford C: Twelve-month test-retest reliability of the structured clinical interview for DSM-III-R personality disorders in cocaine-dependent patients. Compr Psychiatry 36(5):384–389, 1995

Williams ED, Reimherr FW, Marchant BK, Strong RE, et al: Personality disorder in ADHD Part 1: assessment of personality disorder in adult ADHD using data from a clinical trial of OROS methylphenidate. Ann Clin Psychiatry 22(2):84–93, 2010

SCID-5-SPQ and SCID-5-PD Example

This Appendix contains a discussion of the completed sample SCID-5-SPQ and SCID-5-PD for the case of "Nick."

Nick

During the course of a routine physical examination, Nick, a 25-year-old single African American man, unexpectedly started crying and blurted out that he was very depressed, and was thinking about a suicide attempt he had made when he felt this way as a teenager. His doctor referred him for a psychiatric evaluation.

Nick is tall, bearded, muscular, and handsome. He is meticulously dressed in a white suit and has a rose in his lapel. He enters the psychiatrist's office, pauses dramatically, and exclaims, "Aren't roses wonderful this time of year?" When asked why he has come for an evaluation, he replies laughingly that he has done it to appease his family doctor "who seemed worried about me." He has also read a book on psychotherapy, and hopes that "maybe there is someone very special who can understand me. I'd make the most incredible patient." He then takes control of the interview and begins to talk about himself, after first remarking, half jokingly, "I was hoping you would be as attractive as my family doctor."

Nick pulls out of his attaché case a series of newspaper clippings, his résumé, photographs of himself, including some of him with famous people, and a photocopied dollar bill with his face replacing George Washington's. Using these as cues, he begins to tell his story.

He explains that in the last few years he has "discovered" some now-famous actors, one of whom he describes as a "physically perfect teenage heartthrob." He volunteered to coordinate publicity for the actor, and as part of that, posed in a bathing suit in a scene that resembled a famous scene from the actor's hit movie. Nick, imitating the actor's voice, laughingly, and then seriously, describes how he and the actor had similar pasts. Both were rejected by their parents and peers, but overcame this to become popular. When the actor came to town, Nick rented a limousine and showed up at the gala "as a joke," as though he were the star himself. The actor's agent expressed annoyance at

The case of "Nick" has been adapted from Spitzer RL, Gibbon M, Skodol AE, Williams JBW, et al: *DSM-IV-TR Casebook: A Learning Companion to the Diagnostic and Statistical Manual of Mental Disorders, Fourth Edition, Text Revision.* Washington, DC, American Psychiatric Publishing, 2002, pp. 84–85. Used with permission. Copyright © 2002 American Psychiatric Publishing.

The true identity of "Nick" has been disguised. Any details or clinical features that happen to resemble those of an actual person would be a coincidence that we specifically tried to avoid.

what he had done, causing Nick to fly into a rage. When Nick cooled down, he realized that he was "wasting my time promoting others, and that it was time for me to start promoting myself." "Someday," he said, pointing to the picture of the actor, "he will want to be president of my fan club."

Nick has had little previous acting experience of a professional nature, but he is sure that success is "only a question of time." He pulls out some promotional material he has written for his actors and says, "I should write letters to God—He'd love them!" When the psychiatrist is surprised that some materials are signed by a different name than the one Nick has given the receptionist, Nick pulls out a legal document explaining the name change. He has dropped his family name and taken as his new second name his own middle name.

When asked about his love life, Nick says he has no lover, and this is because people are just "superficial." He then displays a newspaper clipping in which he had typeset his and his ex-lover's names in headlines that read: "The relationship is over." More recently he has dated and adored a man with the same first name as his own; but as he became disenchanted, he realized that the man was ugly, and was an embarrassment because he dressed so poorly. Nick then explains that he owns over 100 neckties and about 30 suits, and is proud of how much he spends on "putting myself together." He has no relationships with other homosexual men now, describing them as "only interested in sex." He considers heterosexual men to be "mindless and without aesthetic sense." The only people who have understood him are older men who have suffered as much as he has. "One day, the mindless, happy people who have ignored me will be lining up to see my movies."

Nick's father was very critical, was an alcoholic who was rarely around, and had many affairs. His mother was "like a friend." She was chronically depressed about her husband's affairs and turned to her son, often kissing him good-night, until he was 18, when she started an affair of her own. Nick then felt abandoned and made his suicide gesture. He described a tortured childhood, being picked on by his peers for looking odd, until he began bodybuilding.

At the end of the interview, Nick is referred to an experienced clinician associated with the clinic, who charges a minimal fee ($50/hour), which he can afford. However, Nick requests a referral to someone who would offer him free treatment, seeing no reason for paying anyone because the therapist "would be getting as much out of it as [he] would."

Discussion

Note that the questions whose numbers are circled on the SCID-5-PD correspond to the "YES" answers on the SCID-5-SPQ. Although the SCID-5-PD interview primarily focuses on these circled questions, in most cases SCID-5-PD items corresponding to questions that were not circled should be rated "0" because the corresponding screening questions were answered in the negative. When following up on the circled questions, it is advisable to make a note of the content of the subject's response below the item to allow for a review of the evidence for making the ratings.

Throughout the SCID-5-PD, many items that the subject endorsed on the SCID-5-SPQ eventually end up with a rating of "0" or "1." This is generally due to either the subject misinterpreting the intended meaning of the question or not being able to give sufficient evidence to support a rating of "2." For example, the subject answered "YES" to SCID-5-SPQ Question 19 ("Do you have very high standards about what is right and what is wrong?") because he has very high standards about style and fashion. However, because the question actually inquires about the obsessive-compulsive personality trait of overconscientiousness and inflexibility about matters of morality, ethics, and values, this item (Obsessive-Compulsive Personality Disorder Criterion 4, field code PD21) is rated "0." Similarly, the subject endorsed Question 14 in the SCID-5-SPQ ("When a close relationship ends, do you feel you immediately have to find someone else to take care of you?") because of one breakup after which he went home to his mother. Because this happened on only one occasion, the item in the SCID-5-PD (Dependent Personality Disorder Criterion 7, field code PD15) is finally rated "1."

Note that for both Narcissistic and Borderline Personality Disorders, it was necessary for the interviewer to inquire about all of the criteria, even those for which the subject answered "NO" on the SCID-5-SPQ. Because the subject's presentation during the evaluation was so strongly suggestive of Narcissistic Personality Disorder, during the SCID-5-PD evaluation of Narcissistic Personality Disorder (field codes PD65–PD74), according to the SCID-5-PD rule regarding when to re-ask questions answered "NO" on the SCID-5-SPQ, the interviewer needed to inquire about all of the Narcissistic Personality Disorder items, even though the subject did not endorse all of the corresponding items on the SCID-5-SPQ. Similarly, after limiting the Borderline Personality Disorder inquiry to those items corresponding to "YES" answers on the SCID-5-SPQ, the interviewer was only one item short of making a diagnosis of Borderline Personality Disorder (i.e., only Criteria 1, 2, 4, and 6 were rated "2" and five criteria items are required). Thus, the interviewer needed to inquire about all of the remaining items for which there were "NO" answers on the SCID-5-SPQ in order to ensure that the "NO" answers represented true negatives.

On the SCID-5-PD Summary Score Sheet, the subject is diagnosed as having two Personality Disorders, namely Narcissistic Personality Disorder and Histrionic Personality Disorder, meeting seven criteria items and five criteria items, respectively, for each disorder. In addition, the fact that there are clinically significant features of Borderline Personality Disorder should be noted because a number of the rated items (e.g., unstable and intense relationships, impulsivity, affective instability) were causing clinically significant impairment in his functioning. Finally, the dimensional profile of his ratings indicate predominant elevations in the Cluster B dimensions. (Note that the Antisocial Personality Disorder questions were skipped because of the absence of any symptoms of Conduct Disorder when the subject was a child. If the interviewer was interested in determining a dimensional score for Antisocial Personality Disorder traits, those questions would need to be asked and rated as well).

Sample SCID-5-SPQ and SCID-5-PD for "Nick" begin on next page.

SCID-5-SPQ

Structured Clinical Interview for DSM-5®
Screening Personality Questionnaire

Designed to be used as a screener for the
Structured Clinical Interview for DSM-5® Personality Disorders (SCID-5-PD)

Michael B. First, M.D., Janet B. W. Williams, Ph.D., Lorna Smith Benjamin, Ph.D., and Robert L. Spitzer, M.D.

Your Initials: N A K

Today's Date: O 7 2 4 1 5 PQ1

Study No.: ___ ___ ___ ___ PQ2

ID No.: 1 O 2 3 PQ3

(to be completed by study staff)

Instructions

These questions are about the kind of person you generally are; that is, how you have usually felt or behaved over the past several years. Circle "YES" if the question completely or mostly applies to you or "NO" if the question does not apply to you. If you do not understand a question, leave it blank.

1.	Have you avoided jobs or tasks that involved having to deal with a lot of people?	(NO) YES	PQ4
2.	Do you avoid making friends with people unless you are certain they will like you?	(NO) YES	PQ5
3.	Do you find it hard to be "open" even with people you are close to?	(NO) YES	PQ6
4.	Do you often worry about being criticized or rejected in social situations?	(NO) YES	PQ7
5.	Are you usually quiet when you meet new people?	(NO) YES	PQ8
6.	Do you believe that you're not as good, as smart, or as attractive as most other people?	(NO) YES	PQ9
7.	Are you afraid to do things that might be challenging or to try anything new?	(NO) YES	PQ10
8.	Is it hard for you to make everyday decisions, like what to wear or what to order in a restaurant, without advice and reassurance from others?	NO (YES)	PQ11
9.	Do you depend on other people to handle important areas of your life, such as finances, child care, or living arrangements?	(NO) YES	PQ12
10.	Do you have trouble disagreeing with people even when you think they are wrong?	(NO) YES	PQ13
11.	Do you find it hard to start projects or do things on your own?	(NO) YES	PQ14
12.	Is it so important to you to be taken care of by others that you are willing to do unpleasant or unreasonable things for them?	(NO) YES	PQ15
13.	Do you usually feel uncomfortable when you are by yourself?	(NO) YES	PQ16

14. When a close relationship ends, do you feel you immediately have to find someone else to take care of you?   *NO* (*YES*) | PQ17

15. Do you worry a lot about being left alone to take care of yourself?   (*NO*) *YES* | PQ18

16. Are you the kind of person who spends a lot of time focusing on details, order, or organization, or making lists and schedules?   (*NO*) *YES* | PQ19

17. Do you have trouble finishing things because you spend so much time trying to get them exactly right?   (*NO*) *YES* | PQ20

18. Are you very devoted to your work or to being productive?   (*NO*) *YES* | PQ21

19. Do you have very high standards about what is right and what is wrong?   *NO* (*YES*) | PQ22

20. Do you have trouble throwing things out because they might come in handy someday?   (*NO*) *YES* | PQ23

21. Is it hard for you to work with other people or ask others to do things if they don't agree to do things exactly the way you want?   *NO* (*YES*) | PQ24

22. Is it hard for you to spend money on yourself and other people?   (*NO*) *YES* | PQ25

23. Once you've made plans, is it hard for you to make changes?   (*NO*) *YES* | PQ26

24. Have other people said that you are stubborn?   *NO* (*YES*) | PQ27

25. Do you often get the feeling that people are using you, hurting you, or lying to you?   (*NO*) *YES* | PQ28

26. Are you a very private person who rarely confides in other people?   (*NO*) *YES* | PQ29

27. Do you find that it is best not to let other people know much about you because they will use it against you?   *NO* (*YES*) | PQ30

28. Do you often feel that people are threatening or insulting you by the things they say or do?   (*NO*) *YES* | PQ31

29. Are you the kind of person who holds grudges or takes a long time to forgive people who have insulted or slighted you?   (*NO*) *YES* | PQ32

30.	Are there a lot of people you can't forgive because they did or said something to you a long time ago?	NO	YES	PQ33
31.	Do you often get angry or lash out when someone criticizes or insults you in some way?	NO	YES	PQ34
32.	Have you sometimes suspected that your spouse or partner has been unfaithful?	NO	YES	PQ35
33.	When you are out in public and see people talking, do you often feel that they are talking about you?	NO	YES	PQ36
34.	When you are around people, do you often get the feeling that you are being watched or stared at?	NO	YES	PQ37
35.	Do you often get the feeling that the words to a song or something in a movie or on TV has a special meaning for you in particular?	NO	YES	PQ38
36.	Are you a superstitious person?	NO	YES	PQ39
37.	Have you ever felt that you could make things happen just by making a wish or thinking about them?	NO	YES	PQ40
38.	Have you had personal experiences with the supernatural?	NO	YES	PQ41
39.	Do you believe that you have a "sixth sense" that allows you to know and predict things?	NO	YES	PQ42
40.	Do you often have the feeling that everything is unreal, that you are detached from your body or mind, or that you are an outside observer of your own thoughts or movements?	NO	YES	PQ43
41.	Do you often see things that other people don't see?	NO	YES	PQ44
42.	Do you often hear a voice softly speaking your name?	NO	YES	PQ45
43.	Have you had the sense that some person or force is around you, even though you cannot see anyone?	NO	YES	PQ46
44.	Are there very few people who you're really close to outside of your immediate family?	NO	YES	PQ47

45.	Do you often feel nervous when you are around people you don't know very well?	(NO) YES	PQ48
46.	Is it NOT important to you to have friends or romantic relationships or to be involved with your family?	(NO) YES	PQ49
47.	Would you almost always rather do things alone than with other people?	(NO) YES	PQ50
48.	Do you have little or no interest in having sexual experiences with another person?	(NO) YES	PQ51
49.	Are there really very few things that give you pleasure?	(NO) YES	PQ52
50.	Does it not matter to you what people think of you?	(NO) YES	PQ53
51.	Do you rarely have strong feelings, like being very angry or feeling joyful?	(NO) YES	PQ54
52.	Do you like being the center of attention?	NO (YES)	PQ55
53.	Do you tend to flirt a lot?	NO (YES)	PQ56
54.	Do you often find yourself "coming on" to people?	(NO) YES	PQ57
55.	Do you like to draw attention to yourself by the way you dress or look?	NO (YES)	PQ58
56.	Do you tend to be very dramatic in your actions and speech?	NO (YES)	PQ59
57.	Are you more emotional than most other people, for example, sobbing when you hear a sad story?	(NO) YES	PQ60
58.	Do you often change your mind about things depending on the people you're with or what you have just read or seen on TV?	(NO) YES	PQ61
59.	Do you feel that you are good friends even with people who provide a service, like your plumber, your car mechanic, and your doctor?	(NO) YES	PQ62
60.	Are you more important, more talented, or more successful than most other people?	NO (YES)	PQ63

61.	Have people told you that you have too high an opinion of yourself?	NO **YES**	PQ64
62.	Do you think a lot about the power, success, or recognition that you expect to be yours someday?	NO **YES**	PQ65
63.	Do you think a lot about the perfect romance that will be yours someday?	**NO** YES	PQ66
64.	When you have a problem, do you almost always insist on seeing the top person?	NO **YES**	PQ67
65.	Do you try to spend time with people who are important or influential?	NO **YES**	PQ68
66.	Is it important to you that people pay attention to you or admire you in some way?	NO **YES**	PQ69
67.	Do you feel that you are the kind of person who deserves special treatment, or that other people should automatically do what you want?	NO **YES**	PQ70
68.	Do you often have to put your needs above other people's?	**NO** YES	PQ71
69.	Have others complained that you take advantage of people?	**NO** YES	PQ72
70.	Do you generally feel that other people's needs or feelings are really not your problem?	**NO** YES	PQ73
71.	Do you often find other people's problems to be boring?	**NO** YES	PQ74
72.	Have people complained to you that you don't listen to them or care about their feelings?	**NO** YES	PQ75
73.	When you see someone who is successful, do you feel that you deserve it more than they do?	NO **YES**	PQ76
74.	Do you feel that others are often envious of you?	NO **YES**	PQ77
75.	Do you find that there are very few people who are worth your time and attention?	**NO** YES	PQ78

76. Have other people complained that you act too "high and mighty" or arrogant? (NO) YES | PQ79

77. Have you become frantic when you thought that someone you really cared about was going to leave you? NO (YES) | PQ80

78. Do relationships with people you really care about have lots of extreme ups and downs? NO (YES) | PQ81

79. Does your sense of who you are often change dramatically? (NO) YES | PQ82

80. Are you different with different people or in different situations, so that you sometimes don't know who you really are? (NO) YES | PQ83

81. Have there been lots of sudden changes in your goals, career plans, religious beliefs, and so on? (NO) YES | PQ84

82. Have there been lots of sudden changes in the kinds of friends you have or in your sexual identity? (NO) YES | PQ85

83. Have you often done things impulsively? NO (YES) | PQ86

84. Have you tried to hurt or kill yourself or threatened to do so? NO (YES) | PQ87

85. Have you ever cut, burned, or scratched yourself on purpose? (NO) YES | PQ88

86. Does your mood often change in a single day, based on what's going on in your life? NO (YES) | PQ89

87. Do you often feel empty inside? (NO) YES | PQ90

88. Do you often have temper outbursts or get so angry that you lose control? (NO) YES | PQ91

89. Do you hit people or throw things when you get angry? (NO) YES | PQ92

90. Do even little things get you very angry? (NO) YES | PQ93

91. When you get very upset, do you get suspicious of other people or feel disconnected from your body or that things are unreal? (NO) YES | PQ94

	The following questions apply to things you did before you were 15 years old.			
92.	Before you were 15, did you bully, threaten, or scare other kids?	(NO) YES	PQ95
93.	Before you were 15, did you start fights?	(NO) YES	PQ96
94.	Before you were 15, did you hurt or threaten someone with a weapon, like a bat, brick, broken bottle, a knife, or a gun?	(NO) YES	PQ97
95.	Before you were 15, did you do cruel things to someone that caused him or her physical pain or suffering?	(NO) YES	PQ98
96.	Before you were 15, did you hurt animals on purpose?	(NO) YES	PQ99
97.	Before you were 15, did you mug, rob, or forcibly take something from someone by threatening him or her?	(NO) YES	PQ100
98.	Before you were 15, did you force someone to do something sexual?	(NO) YES	PQ101
99.	Before you were 15, did you set fires?	(NO) YES	PQ102
100.	Before you were 15, did you deliberately destroy things that weren't yours?	(NO) YES	PQ103
101.	Before you were 15, did you break into houses, other buildings, or cars?	(NO) YES	PQ104
102.	Before you were 15, did you lie a lot or con other people to get something you wanted or to get out of doing something?	(NO) YES	PQ105
103.	Before you were 15, did you sometimes shoplift, steal something, or forge someone's signature for money?	(NO) YES	PQ106
104.	Before you were 15, did you run away and stay away overnight?	(NO) YES	PG107

	The following two questions apply to things you did before you were 13 years old.			
105.	Before you were 13, did you often stay out very late, long after the time you were supposed to be home?	(NO) YES	PQ108
106.	Before you were 13, did you often skip school?	(NO) YES	PQ109

SCID-5-PD

STRUCTURED CLINICAL INTERVIEW
FOR DSM-5® PERSONALITY DISORDERS

Michael B. First, M.D.
Professor of Clinical Psychiatry, Columbia University, and Research Psychiatrist,
Division of Clinical Phenomenology, New York State Psychiatric Institute, New York, New York

Janet B. W. Williams, Ph.D.
Professor Emerita of Clinical Psychiatric Social Work (in Psychiatry and in Neurology), Columbia University,
and Research Scientist and Deputy Chief, Biometrics Research Department (Retired),
New York State Psychiatric Institute, New York, New York; and
Senior Vice President of Global Science, MedAvante, Inc., Hamilton, New Jersey

Lorna Smith Benjamin, Ph.D.
Adjunct Professor of Psychiatry and Professor Emerita of Psychology,
University of Utah, Salt Lake City, Utah

Robert L. Spitzer, M.D.
Professor Emeritus of Psychiatry, Columbia University, and
Research Scientist and Chief, Biometrics Research Department (Retired),
New York State Psychiatric Institute, New York, New York

Patient: _Nick_____		Date of Interview:	_07_	_28_	_15_
			month	day	year
Clinician: _Dr. First_____					

SCID-5-PD DIAGNOSTIC SUMMARY SCORE SHEET

Overall quality and completeness of information: 1 = Poor   2 = Fair   (3 = Good)   4 = Excellent

Duration of interview (minutes) _0 3 0_

ICD-10-CM code	Personality Disorder	Categorical criteria met?*	If criteria not met, are there clinically significant features?***	Dimensional profile Based on sum of ratings (0, 1, and 2)
Cluster C Personality Disorders				
F60.6	Avoidant	(NO) YES (4 of 7) (page 8)	(NO) YES (pages 7–8)	(0) 1 2 3 4 5 6 7 8 9 10 11 12 13 14
F60.7	Dependent	(NO) YES (5 of 8) (page 11)	(NO) YES (pages 9–11)	0 1 (2) 3 4 5 6 7 8 9 10 11 12 13 14 15 16
F60.5	Obsessive-Compulsive	(NO) YES (4 of 8) (page 14)	(NO) YES (pages 12–14)	0 1 (2) 3 4 5 6 7 8 9 10 11 12 13 14 15 16
Cluster A Personality Disorders				
F60.0	Paranoid	(NO) YES (4 of 7 and Crit B**) (page 17)	NO YES (pages 15–17)	0 (1) 2 3 4 5 6 7 8 9 10 11 12 13 14
F21	Schizotypal	(NO) YES (5 of 9 and Crit B**) (page 21)	NO YES (pages 18–21)	(0) 1 2 3 4 5 6 7 8 9 10 11 12 13 14 15 16 17 18
F60.1	Schizoid	(NO) YES (4 of 7 and Crit B**) (page 24)	NO YES (pages 22–24)	(0) 1 2 3 4 5 6 7 8 9 10 11 12 13 14
Cluster B Personality Disorders				
F60.4	Histrionic	NO (YES) (5 of 8) (page 26)	NO YES (pages 25–26)	0 1 2 3 4 5 6 7 8 9 (10) 11 12 13 14 15 16
F60.81	Narcissistic	NO (YES) (5 of 9) (page 29)	NO YES (pages 27–29)	0 1 2 3 4 5 6 7 8 9 10 11 12 13 (14) 15 16 17 18
F60.3	Borderline	(NO) YES (5 of 9) (page 33)	(NO) YES (pages 30–33)	0 1 2 3 4 5 6 7 8 (9) 10 11 12 13 14 15 16 17 18
F60.2	Antisocial	(NO) YES (3 of 7 [page 39] and 2+ Conduct sx [page 36])	NO YES (pages 34–39)	0 1 2 3 4 5 6 7 8 9 10 11 12 13 14
Other Specified Personality Disorder				
F60.89	Other Specified	(NO) YES (page 40)	—	If non-DSM-5 personality disorder, indicate name:

*Page numbers refer to the SCID-5-PD pages where the categorical diagnosis of the disorder is made.

**Criterion B: Does not occur exclusively during the course of Schizophrenia, a Bipolar Disorder or Depressive Disorder With Psychotic Features, another Psychotic Disorder, or Autism Spectrum Disorder. (*Note:* Autism Spectrum Disorder is not included among the excluded conditions in Paranoid Personality Disorder.)

***Clinically significant features* as described in Criterion C, "General Personality Disorder Criteria That Should Be Considered When Making a Rating of '2'": The features have a negative impact on the person's social interactions, ability to form and maintain close relationships, and/or the ability to function effectively at work, school, or home.

PRINCIPAL PERSONALITY DISORDER DIAGNOSIS (i.e., the Personality Disorder that is, or should be, the main focus of clinical attention):

Enter ICD-10-CM code number from left of diagnosis above: F _60.81_
(Note: Leave blank if no Personality Disorder.)

GENERAL OVERVIEW

NOTE: IF SCID-5 OVERVIEW HAS ALREADY BEEN COMPLETED, SKIP TO
OVERVIEW FOR ASSESSMENT OF PERSONALITY DISORDERS, *PAGE 4.*

I'm going to start by asking you about problems or difficulties you may have had, and I'll be making some notes as we go along. Do you have any questions before we begin?

NOTE: Any current suicidal thoughts, plans, or actions should be thoroughly assessed by the clinician and action taken if necessary.

Demographic Data

How old are you? 25

Are you married? No

　　IF NO: **Do you live with someone as if you are married?** No

　　　　IF NO: **Were you ever married?** No

How long have you been (MARITAL STATUS)?

IF EVER MARRIED: **How many times have you been married?**

Do you have any children? No

　　IF YES: **How many? (What are their ages?)**

With whom do you live? (How many children under the age of 18 live in your household?) By myself

---

Education and Work History

How far did you go in school? Graduated College

IF SUBJECT FAILED TO COMPLETE A PROGRAM IN WHICH HE OR SHE WAS ENROLLED: **Why did you leave?**

What kind of work do you do? (Do you work outside of your home?) Public Relations, Talent Agent

Have you always done that kind of work? Yes

　　IF NO: **What other kind of work have you done in the past?**

What's the longest you've worked at one place? *8 months*

Are you currently employed (getting paid)? *Yes, working as a barista at Starbucks temporarily until my business gets established*

    IF NO: **Why not?**

IF UNKNOWN: **Has there ever been a period of time when you were unable to work or go to school?**

    IF YES: **Why was that?**

Have you ever been arrested, involved in a lawsuit, or had other legal trouble? *No*

Current and Past Periods of Psychopathology

Have you ever seen anybody for emotional or psychiatric problems? *Yes*

    IF YES: **What was that for? (What treatment[s] did you get? Any medications? When was that?)** *I saw a psychologist three times after I took an overdose of NyQuil after I found out my mother was having an affair when I was 18*

    IF NO: **Was there ever a time when you, or someone else, thought you should see someone because of the way you were feeling or acting? (Tell me more.)**

Have you ever seen anybody for problems with alcohol or drugs? *No*

    IF YES: **What was that for? (What treatment[s] did you get? Any medications? When was that?)**

Have you ever attended a self-help group, like Alcoholics Anonymous, Gamblers Anonymous, or Overeaters Anonymous? *No*

    IF YES: **What was that for? When was that?**

Have you used a lot of alcohol or taken a lot of drugs for much of the time in your life? Tell me about that. *Drinking on the weekends, ecstasy at parties*

Thinking back over your whole life, when were you the most upset? (Tell me about that. What was that like? How were you feeling?) *when my first boyfriend broke up with me at age 22, I was devastated*

OVERVIEW FOR ASSESSMENT OF PERSONALITY DISORDERS

Now I am going to ask you some questions about the kind of person you are—that is, how you generally have felt or behaved.

IF A CIRCUMSCRIBED OR EPISODIC NON–PERSONALITY DISORDER HAS BEEN PRESENT: **I know that there have been times when you have been** (SXS OF DISORDER). **I am not talking about those times, and you should try to think of how you usually are when you are not** (SXS). **Do you have any questions about this?**

How would you describe yourself as a person before (SXS OF DISORDER)**?**

IF CAN'T ANSWER, MOVE ON.

How do you think other people would describe you as a person before (SXS OF DISORDER)**?**

Who have been the important people in your life?

    IF MENTIONS ONLY FAMILY: **What about friends?**

How have you gotten along with them?

Do you think that the usual way that you react to things or behave with people has caused you problems with anyone? (At home? At school? At work?) (In what way?)

How successful would you say you are at getting the things you want in life, like having a satisfying relationship, a fulfilling career, or close friends?

Not yet. It's just a matter of time until I become a star.

How do you spend your free time?

Who do you spend it with?

If you could change your personality in some ways, how would you want to be different?

IF SCID-5-SPQ HAS BEEN COMPLETED: **Now I want to go over the questions you said "YES" to on the questionnaire.**

IF SCID-5-SPQ HAS NOT BEEN COMPLETED: **Now I want to ask you some more specific questions.**

GENERAL PERSONALITY DISORDER CRITERIA THAT SHOULD BE CONSIDERED WHEN MAKING A RATING OF "2"

Review and consider the following general personality disorder criteria when determining whether a particular Personality Disorder criterion warrants a rating of "2" (Threshold).

A. An enduring pattern of inner experience and behavior that deviates markedly from the expectations of the individual's culture. A Personality Disorder criterion must be at the extreme end of that continuum for it to warrant a rating of "2."

> **What is that like?**
> **Give me some examples.**
> **Do you think you are more this way than most people you know?**

B. The enduring pattern is inflexible and pervasive across a broad range of personal and social situations. A Personality Disorder criterion should be expressed consistently across most situations and not be restricted to a single interpersonal relationship, situation, or role.

> **Does this happen in a lot of different situations?**
> **Does this happen with a lot of different people?**

C. The enduring pattern leads to clinically significant distress or impairment in social, occupational, or other important areas of functioning. A Personality Disorder criterion should have a negative impact on the person's social interactions, ability to form and maintain close relationships, and/or the ability to function effectively at work, school, or home.

> **What problems has this caused for you?**
> **Has this affected your relationships or your interactions with other people? (How about your family, romantic partner, or friends?)**
> **Has this affected your work/school?**
> **Has it bothered other people?**

D. The pattern is stable and of long duration, and its onset can be traced back at least to adolescence or early adulthood. A Personality Disorder criterion must have been frequently present over a period of at least the last 5 years and there must be evidence of the trait going back as far as the person's late teens or early 20s.

> **Have you been this way for a long time?**
> **How often does this happen?**
> **When can you first remember (feeling/acting) this way? (Do you remember a period of time when you didn't feel this way?)**

E. The enduring pattern is not better explained as a manifestation or consequence of another mental disorder. If another mental disorder has been present, the course of the Personality Disorder criterion must occur independently of the other mental disorder (e.g., onset is prior to the other mental disorder or is significant at times the other mental disorder is not prominent).

> *IF THERE IS EVIDENCE OF ANOTHER MENTAL DISORDER WITH SYMPTOMS THAT RESEMBLE THE PERSONALITY ITEM IN QUESTION:* **Does this happen only when you are having** (SXS OF MENTAL DISORDER)**?**

F. The enduring pattern is not attributable to the physiological effects of a substance (e.g., a drug of abuse, a medication) or another medical condition (e.g., head trauma). If there is a history of chronic substance use, the Personality Disorder criterion is not better explained as a manifestation of chronic recurrent substance intoxication or withdrawal and is not exclusively associated with activities in the service of sustaining substance use (e.g., antisocial behavior). If a general medical condition (GMC) is present, the Personality Disorder criterion is not better explained as a direct physiological consequence of the GMC.

> *IF THERE IS EVIDENCE OF PROLONGED EXCESSIVE ALCOHOL OR DRUG USE THAT RESULTS IN SYMPTOMS THAT RESEMBLE THE PERSONALITY ITEM IN QUESTION:* **Does this happen only when you are drunk or high or withdrawing from alcohol or drugs? Does this happen only when you are trying to get alcohol or drugs?**

> *IF THERE IS EVIDENCE OF A GMC THAT RESULTS IN SYMPTOMS THAT RESEMBLE THE PERSONALITY ITEM IN QUESTION:* **Were you like that before** (ONSET OF GMC)**?**

ASSESSMENT OF DSM-5 PERSONALITY DISORDERS

AVOIDANT PERSONALITY DISORDER	AVOIDANT PERSONALITY DISORDER CRITERIA

*A pervasive pattern of social inhibition, feelings of inadequacy, and hypersensitivity to negative evaluation, beginning by early adulthood and present in a variety of contexts, as indicated by **four** (or more) of the following:*

1. **You've said that you have** *[Have you]* **avoided jobs or tasks that involved having to deal with a lot of people.**

   Give me some examples.

   What was the reason that you avoided these (JOBS OR TASKS)**? (Is it because you just don't like to be around people, or is it because you are afraid of being criticized or rejected?)**

   1. Avoids occupational activities that involve significant interpersonal contact because of fears of criticism, disapproval, or rejection.

      2 = at least two examples

   ? ⓪ 1 2   PD1

2. **You've said that** *[Do]* **you avoid making friends with people unless you are certain they will like you.**

   Do you avoid joining in group activities unless you are sure that you will be welcomed and accepted?

   If you don't know whether someone likes you, would you ever make the first move?

   2. Is unwilling to get involved with people unless certain of being liked.

      2 = almost never takes the initiative in becoming involved in a social relationship

   ? ⓪ 1 2   PD2

3. **You've said that** *[Do]* **you find it hard to be "open" even with people you are close to.**

   Why is this? (Are you afraid of being made fun of or embarrassed?)

   3. Shows restraint within intimate relationships because of the fear of being shamed or ridiculed.

      2 = true for almost all relationships

   ? ⓪ 1 2   PD3

? = Inadequate information   0 = Absent   1 = Subthreshold   2 = Threshold

4.   **You've said that** *[Do]* **you often worry about being criticized or rejected in social situations. Give me some examples.**

     Do you spend a lot of time worrying about this?

4. Is preoccupied with being criticized or rejected in social situations. *2 = a lot of time spent worrying about social situations*	? (0) 1 2			PD4

5.   **You've said that you're** *[Are you]* **usually quiet when you meet new people.**

     Why is that?

     (Is it because you feel in some way inadequate or not good enough?)

5. Is inhibited in new interpersonal situations because of feelings of inadequacy.

     2 = acknowledges trait and many examples   ? (0) 1 2   PD5

6.   **You've said that** *[Do]* **you believe that you're not as good, as smart, or as attractive as most other people.**

     Tell me about that.

6. Views self as socially inept, personally unappealing, or inferior to others.

     2 = acknowledges belief   ? (0) 1 2   PD6

7.   **You've said that you're** *[Are you]* **afraid to do things that might be challenging or to try anything new.**

     Is that because you are afraid of being embarrassed?

     Give me some examples.

7. Is unusually reluctant to take personal risks or to engage in any new activities because they may prove embarrassing.

     2 = several examples of avoiding activities because of fear of embarrassment   ? (0) 1 2   PD7

AT LEAST FOUR CRITERIA (1–7) ARE RATED "2"   (NO)   YES   PD8

> Avoidant Personality Disorder

? = Inadequate information   0 = Absent   1 = Subthreshold   2 = Threshold

<u>**DEPENDENT PERSONALITY DISORDER**</u>   <u>**DEPENDENT PERSONALITY DISORDER CRITERIA**</u>

*A pervasive and excessive need to be taken care of that leads to submissive and clinging behavior and fears of separation, beginning by early adulthood and present in a variety of contexts, as indicated by **five** (or more) of the following:*

(8.) **You've said that it is** *[Is it]* **hard for you** *to* **make everyday decisions, like what to wear or what to order in a restaurant, without advice and reassurance from others.** **Can you give me some examples of the kinds of decisions you would ask for advice or reassurance about?** **(Does this happen most of the time?)**	1. Has difficulty making everyday decisions without an excessive amount of advice and reassurance from others. *2 = several examples* *Sometimes - what to wear* (handwritten)	? 0 (1) 2	PD9
9. **You've said that you** *[Do you]* **depend on other people to handle important areas of your life, such as finances, child care, or living arrangements.** **Give me some examples. (Is this more than just getting advice from people?)** **(Has this happened with MOST important areas of your life?)**	2. Needs others to assume responsibility for most major areas of his or her life. *[Note: Do not include merely getting advice from others or subculturally expected behavior.]* *2 = several examples*	? (0) 1 2	PD10
10. **You've said that** *[Do]* **you have trouble disagreeing with people even when you think they are wrong.** **Give me some examples of when that has happened.** **What are you afraid would happen if you disagree?**	3. Has difficulty expressing disagreement with others because of fear of loss of support or approval. (**Note:** Do not include realistic fears of retribution.) *2 = acknowledges trait or several examples*	? (0) 1 2	PD11

11.	**You've said** *[Do]* **you find it hard to start projects or do things on your own.** **Give me some examples.** **Why is that? (Is this because you are not sure you can do it right?)** **(Can you do it as long as there is someone there to help you?)**	4.	Has difficulty initiating projects or doing things on his or her own (because of a lack of self-confidence in judgment or abilities rather than a lack of motivation or energy). *2 = acknowledges trait*	?	⓪	1	2	PD12

12.	**You've said that it is** *[Is it]* **so important to you to be taken care of by others that you are willing to do unpleasant or unreasonable things for them.** **Give me some examples of these kinds of things.**	5.	Goes to excessive lengths to obtain nurturance and support from others, to the point of volunteering to do things that are unpleasant. *[Note: Do not include behavior intended to achieve goals other than being liked, such as job advancement.]* *2 = acknowledges trait and at least one example*	?	⓪	1	2	PD13

13.	**You've said that** *[Do]* **you usually feel uncomfortable when you are by yourself.** **Why is that? (Is it because you need someone to take care of you?)**	6.	Feels uncomfortable or helpless when alone because of exaggerated fears of being unable to care for himself or herself. *2 = acknowledges trait*	?	⓪	1	2	PD14

(14.)	**You've said that when a close relationship ends, you** *[When a close relationship ends, do you]* **feel you immediately have to find someone else to take care of you.** **Tell me about that.** **(Have you reacted this way most of the time when close relationships have ended?)**	7.	Urgently seeks another relationship as a source of care and support when a close relationship ends. *2 = happens when most close relationships end* With first lover went home to live with mother	?	0	①	2	PD15

? = Inadequate information   0 = Absent   1 = Subthreshold   2 = Threshold

15. **You've said that** *[Do]* **you worry a lot about being left alone to take care of yourself.**

What makes you think that you are going to be left alone to take care of yourself? (How realistic is this fear?)

How much do you worry about this?

8. Is unrealistically preoccupied with fears of being left to take care of himself or herself.

    2 = worry is excessive and unrealistic

    ?   ⓪   1   2   PD16

AT LEAST FIVE CRITERIA (1–8) ARE RATED "2"   (NO)   YES   PD17

→ Dependent Personality Disorder

? = Inadequate information   0 = Absent   1 = Subthreshold   2 = Threshold

OBSESSIVE-COMPULSIVE PERSONALITY DISORDER	OBSESSIVE-COMPULSIVE PERSONALITY DISORDER CRITERIA					

*A pervasive pattern of preoccupation with orderliness, perfectionism, and mental and interpersonal control, at the expense of flexibility, openness, and efficiency, beginning by early adulthood and present in a variety of contexts, as indicated by **four** (or more) of the following:*

16. **You've said that you are** *[Are you]* **the kind of person who spends a lot of time focusing on details, order, or organization, or making lists and schedules.**

    Tell me about that.

    Do you spend so much time doing this that the point of what you were trying to do gets lost? (For example, you spend so much time preparing a list of things you have to do that you don't have enough time to get them done.)

    1. Is preoccupied with details, rules, lists, order, organization, or schedules to the extent that the major point of the activity is lost.

       2 = acknowledges trait and at least one example

       ? (0) 1 2   PD18

17. **You've said that** *[Do]* **you have trouble finishing things because you spend so much time trying to get them exactly right.**

    Give me some examples.

    (How often does this happen?)

    2. Shows perfectionism that interferes with task completion (e.g., is unable to complete a project because his or her own overly strict standards are not met).

       2 = several examples of tasks not completed or significantly delayed because of perfectionism

       ? (0) 1 2   PD19

18. **You've said that you are** *[Are you]* **very devoted to your work or to being productive.**

    Are you so devoted that you rarely get to spend time with friends, go on vacation, or do things just for fun?

    (When you do take time off, do you always take work along because you can't stand to "waste time"?)

    3. Is excessively devoted to work and productivity to the exclusion of leisure activities and friendships (not accounted for by obvious economic necessity).

       [Note: Also not accounted for by temporary job requirements.]

       2 = acknowledges trait or has been told by other people

       ? (0) 1 2   PD20

? = Inadequate information   0 = Absent   1 = Subthreshold   2 = Threshold

		?	0	1	2	

19. You've said that *[Do]* you have very high standards about what is right and what is wrong.

Give me some examples of your high standards.

(Do you follow rules to the letter of the law, no matter what? Do you insist that others also follow the rules? Can you give me some examples?)

IF GIVES RELIGIOUS EXAMPLE:
Are you stricter than other people who share your religious views?

4. Is overconscientious, scrupulous, and inflexible about matters of morality, ethics, or values (not accounted for by cultural or religious identification).

2 = several examples of holding self or others to rigidly high moral standards

About how I dress and look.

? (0) 1 2   PD21

20. You've said that *[Do]* you have trouble throwing things out because they might come in handy someday.

Give me some examples of things that you're unable to throw out. (What about things that are worn out or worthless?)

5. Is unable to discard worn-out or worthless objects even when they have no sentimental value.

2 = several examples of worn-out or worthless objects

? (0) 1 2   PD22

21. You've said that it is *[Is it]* hard for you to work with other people or ask others to do things if they don't agree to do things exactly the way you want.

Tell me about that. (Does this happen often?)

(Do you often end up doing things yourself to make sure they are done right?)

6. Is reluctant to delegate tasks or to work with others unless they submit to exactly his or her way of doing things.

2 = acknowledges trait and at least one example

I want things to look just right. E.g., dinner parties. I have to do it all myself.

? 0 1 (2)   PD23

22. You've said that it is *[Is it]* hard for you to spend money on yourself and other people.

Why? (Is this because you're worried about not having enough in the future when you might really need it? What might you need it for?)

Has anyone said that you are "stingy" or "miserly"?

7. Adopts a miserly spending style toward both self and others; money is viewed as something to be hoarded for future catastrophes.

2 = acknowledges trait and at least one example

? (0) 1 2   PD24

? = Inadequate information   0 = Absent   1 = Subthreshold   2 = Threshold

23. **You've said that once you've made plans, it is** [Once you've made plans, is it] **hard for you to make changes.**

Tell me about that.

(Are you so concerned about having things done the one "correct" way that you have trouble going along with anyone else's ideas? Tell me about that.)

24. **You've said that other people have** [Have other people] **said that you are stubborn.**

Tell me about that.

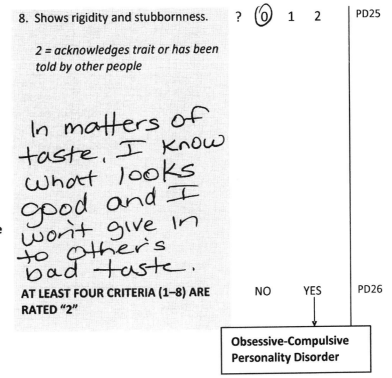

8. Shows rigidity and stubbornness.   ? ⓪ 1 2   PD25

   2 = acknowledges trait or has been told by other people

In matters of taste, I know what looks good and I won't give in to other's bad taste.

AT LEAST FOUR CRITERIA (1–8) ARE RATED "2"   NO   YES   PD26

Obsessive-Compulsive Personality Disorder

? = Inadequate information   0 = Absent   1 = Subthreshold   2 = Threshold

PARANOID PERSONALITY DISORDER	PARANOID PERSONALITY DISORDER CRITERIA					

A. *A pervasive distrust and suspiciousness of others such that their motives are interpreted as malevolent, beginning by early adulthood and present in a variety of contexts, as indicated by* **four** *(or more) of the following:*

25. **You've said that** *[Do]* **you often get the feeling that people are using you, hurting you, or lying to you.**

    What makes you think that?

1. Suspects, without sufficient basis, that others are exploiting, harming, or deceiving him or her.

   2 = acknowledges trait and at least one example

   ? ⓪ 1 2   PD27

26. **You've said that you are** *[Are you]* **a very private person who rarely confides in other people.**

    Is it because you don't trust your friends or the people you work with? Why don't you trust them?

    Do you spend a lot of time thinking about this?

2. Is preoccupied with unjustified doubts about the loyalty or trustworthiness of friends or associates.

   2 = acknowledges preoccupation with trustworthiness or loyalty of other people

   ? ⓪ 1 2   PD28

(27.) **You've said that** *[Do]* **you find that it is best not to let other people know much about you because they will use it against you.**

    When has this happened?

    Tell me about that.

3. Is reluctant to confide in others because of unwarranted fear that the information will be used maliciously against him or her.

   2 = acknowledges trait

   ? 0 ① 2   PD29

   Not with friends but have to be careful with show biz types, everyone out for themselves

28. **You've said that** *[Do]* **you often feel that people are threatening or insulting you by the things they say or do.**

    Tell me about that.

4. Reads hidden demeaning or threatening meanings into benign remarks or events.

   2 = acknowledges trait and at least one example of misinterpreting a benign remark or action

   ? ⓪ 1 2   PD30

? = Inadequate information   0 = Absent   1 = Subthreshold   2 = Threshold

29.	You've said that you're *[Are you]* the kind of person who holds grudges or takes a long time to forgive people who have insulted or slighted you. Tell me about that.	5. Persistently bears grudges (i.e., is unforgiving of insults, injuries, or slights). *2 = acknowledges trait and at least one example*	?	(0)	1	2	PD31

30.	You've said that there are *[Are there]* a lot of people you can't forgive because they did or said something to you a long time ago. Tell me about that.						

(31.)	You've said that *[Do]* you often get angry or lash out when someone criticizes or insults you in some way. Give me some examples. (Do others say that you often take offense too easily?)	6. Perceives attacks on his or her character or reputation that are not apparent to others and is quick to react angrily or to counterattack. *I have a temper. E.g., I was really pissed when* *2 = acknowledges trait and at least one example* ↓ *that agent told me to get out.*	?	(0)	1	2	PD32

(32.)	You've said that you have *[Have you]* sometimes suspected that your spouse or partner has been unfaithful. Tell me about that. (What clues did you have? What did you do about it? Were you right?)	7. Has recurrent suspicions, without justification, regarding fidelity of spouse or sexual partner. *2 = examples of unjustified suspicions with several partners or on several occasions with the same partner OR acknowledges trait* He was screwing around with everyone.	?	(0)	1	2	PD33

? = Inadequate information   0 = Absent   1 = Subthreshold   2 = Threshold

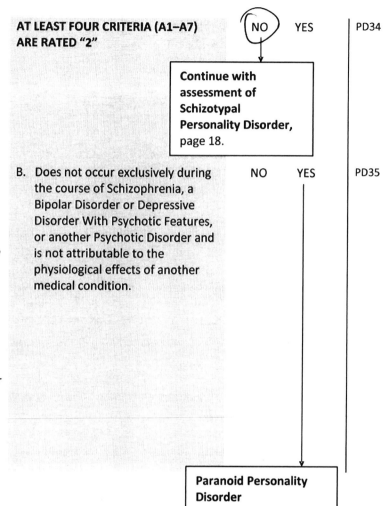

AT LEAST FOUR CRITERIA (A1–A7)   NO   YES   PD34
ARE RATED "2"

Continue with
assessment of
Schizotypal
Personality Disorder,
page 18.

IF THERE IS EVIDENCE OF A PSYCHOTIC DISORDER: **Does this happen only when you are having (SXS OF PSYCHOTIC DISORDER)?**

IF THERE IS EVIDENCE OF PROLONGED EXCESSIVE ALCOHOL OR DRUG USE THAT RESULTS IN SYMPTOMS THAT RESEMBLE PARANOID PD: **Does this happen only when you are drunk or high or withdrawing from alcohol or drugs?**

IF THERE IS EVIDENCE OF A GMC THAT CAUSES SYMPTOMS THAT RESEMBLE PARANOID PD: **Were you like that before (ONSET OF GMC)?**

B. Does not occur exclusively during   NO   YES   PD35
the course of Schizophrenia, a
Bipolar Disorder or Depressive
Disorder With Psychotic Features,
or another Psychotic Disorder and
is not attributable to the
physiological effects of another
medical condition.

Paranoid Personality Disorder

? = Inadequate information   0 = Absent   1 = Subthreshold   2 = Threshold

<table>
<tr><td>

SCHIZOTYPAL PERSONALITY DISORDER

</td><td>

SCHIZOTYPAL PERSONALITY DISORDER CRITERIA

</td></tr>
</table>

SCHIZOTYPAL PERSONALITY DISORDER

SCHIZOTYPAL PERSONALITY DISORDER CRITERIA

A. A pervasive pattern of social and interpersonal deficits marked by acute discomfort with, and reduced capacity for, close relationships as well as by cognitive or perceptual distortions and eccentricities of behavior, beginning by early adulthood and present in a variety of contexts, as indicated by **five** (or more) of the following:

(33.) You've said that when you are out in public and see people talking, *[When you are out in public and see people talking, do]* you often feel that they are talking about you.

Tell me more about this.

1. Ideas of reference (excluding delusions of reference).   ? (0) 1 2   PD36

2 = several examples

People notice me because I'm good looking and dress stylishly.

(34.) You've said that when you are around people, you *[When you are around people, do you]* often get the feeling that you are being watched or stared at.

Tell me more about this.

35. You've said that you *[Do you]* often get the feeling that the words to a song or something in a movie or on TV has a special meaning for you in particular.

Tell me more about this.

? = Inadequate information   0 = Absent   1 = Subthreshold   2 = Threshold

36.	You've said that you are *[Are you]* a superstitious person. What are some of your superstitions? How have they affected what you say or do? Do you know other people who do these things?	2.	Odd beliefs or magical thinking that influences behavior and is inconsistent with subcultural norms (e.g., superstitiousness, belief in clairvoyance, telepathy, or "sixth sense"; in children and adolescents, bizarre fantasies or preoccupations).	? ⓪ 1 2		PD37
37.	You've said that you have *[Have you ever]* felt that you could make things happen just by making a wish or thinking about them. Tell me about that. (How did it affect you?)		*2 = several examples of such phenomena that influenced behavior and are inconsistent with subcultural norms*			
38.	You've said that you have *[Have you]* had personal experiences with the supernatural. Tell me about that. (How did it affect you?)					
39.	You've said that you *[Do you]* believe that you have a "sixth sense" that allows you to know and predict things. Tell me about that. (How does it affect you?)					

? = Inadequate information   0 = Absent   1 = Subthreshold   2 = Threshold

40.	You've said that you *[Do you]* often have the feeling that everything is unreal, that you are detached from your body or mind, or that you are an outside observer of your own thoughts or movements. Give me some examples. (Were you drinking or taking drugs at the time?)	3. Unusual perceptual experiences, including bodily illusions. *2 = several examples of unusual perceptual experiences not due to substance use*	? ⓪ 1 2	PD38
41.	You've said that *[Do]* you often see things that other people don't see. Give me some examples. (Were you drinking or taking drugs at the time?)			
42.	You've said that you *[Do you]* often hear a voice softly speaking your name. Tell me more about that. (Were you drinking or taking drugs at the time?)			
43.	You've said that you have *[Have you]* had the sense that some person or force is around you, even though you cannot see anyone. Tell me more about that. (Were you drinking or taking drugs at the time?)			
	OBSERVED DURING INTERVIEW	4. Odd thinking and speech (e.g., vague, circumstantial, metaphorical, overelaborate, or stereotyped).	? ⓪ 1 2	PD39
	IF ANY OF PARANOID PD CRITERIA A1, A2, A3, A4, OR A7 ARE RATED "2"	5. Suspiciousness or paranoid ideation.	? ⓪ 1 2	PD40
	OBSERVED DURING INTERVIEW	6. Inappropriate or constricted affect.	? ⓪ 1 2	PD41
	OBSERVED DURING INTERVIEW	7. Behavior or appearance that is odd, eccentric, or peculiar.	? ⓪ 1 2	PD42

? = Inadequate information   0 = Absent   1 = Subthreshold   2 = Threshold

44. **You've said that there are** *[Are there]* **very few people who you're really close to outside of your immediate family.** **How many close friends do you have?**	8. Lack of close friends or confidants other than first-degree relatives. *2 = no close friends (other than first-degree relatives)*	? ⓪ 1 2	PD43
45. **You've said that** *[Do]* **you often feel nervous when you are around people you don't know very well. What are you nervous about?** **Is it because you are worried about being taken advantage of or hurt in some way rather than being rejected or criticized?** **(Are you still anxious even after you've known them for a while?)**	9. Excessive social anxiety that does not diminish with familiarity and tends to be associated with paranoid fears rather than negative judgments about self. *2 = acknowledges excessive anxiety that does not diminish with familiarity related to suspiciousness about other people's motives*	? ⓪ 1 2	PD44
	AT LEAST FIVE CRITERIA (A1–A9) ARE RATED "2"	ⓃⓄ YES	PD45

> **Continue with assessment of Schizoid Personality Disorder**, page 22.

IF THERE IS EVIDENCE OF A PSYCHOTIC DISORDER: **Does this happen only when you are having** (SXS OF PSYCHOTIC DISORDER)**?** *IF THERE IS EVIDENCE OF PROLONGED EXCESSIVE ALCOHOL OR DRUG USE THAT RESULTS IN SYMPTOMS THAT RESEMBLE SCHIZOTYPAL PD:* **Does this happen only when you are drunk or high or withdrawing from alcohol or drugs?** *IF THERE IS EVIDENCE OF A GMC THAT CAUSES SYMPTOMS THAT RESEMBLE SCHIZOTYPAL PD:* **Were you like that before** (ONSET OF GMC)**?**	B. Does not occur exclusively during the course of Schizophrenia, a Bipolar Disorder or Depressive Disorder With Psychotic Features, another Psychotic Disorder, or Autism Spectrum Disorder. *[Note: This criterion should be rated "NO" if there is a preexisting diagnosis of Autism Spectrum Disorder.]*	ⓃⓄ YES	PD46

> **Schizotypal Personality Disorder**

SCHIZOID PERSONALITY DISORDER	SCHIZOID PERSONALITY DISORDER CRITERIA					
	A. A pervasive pattern of detachment from social relationships and a restricted range of expression of emotions in interpersonal settings, beginning by early adulthood and present in a variety of contexts, as indicated by **four** (or more) of the following:					
46. **You've said that it is** [Is it] **NOT important to you to have friends or romantic relationships or to be involved with your family.** **Tell me more about that.**	1. Neither desires nor enjoys close relationships, including being part of a family. 2 = acknowledges trait	?	⓪	1	2	PD47
47. **You've said that you would** [Would you] **almost always rather do things alone than with other people.** **(Is that true both at work and during your free time?)**	2. Almost always chooses solitary activities. 2 = acknowledges trait	?	⓪	1	2	PD48
48. **You've said that** [Do] **you have little or no interest in having sexual experiences with another person.** **Tell me more about that.**	3. Has little, if any, interest in having sexual experiences with another person. 2 = acknowledges trait	?	⓪	1	2	PD49
49. **You've said that there are** [Are there] **really very few things that give you pleasure.** **Tell me about that.** **(What about physical things like eating a good meal or having sex?)**	4. Takes pleasure in few, if any, activities. [Note: Absence of pleasure especially applies to sensory, bodily, and interpersonal experiences.] 2 = acknowledges trait	?	⓪	1	2	PD50

? = Inadequate information   0 = Absent   1 = Subthreshold   2 = Threshold

PREVIOUSLY RATED IN **CRITERION A8** *FOR SCHIZOTYPAL PD.* *IF NOT PREVIOUSLY RATED THERE, USE THE FOLLOWING QUESTION, CORRESPONDING TO* **QUESTION 44** *ON THE SCID-5-SPQ.* **You've said that there are** *[Are there]* **very few people who you're really close to outside of your immediate family.** **How many close friends do you have?**	5. Lacks close friends or confidants other than first-degree relatives. *2 = no close friends (other than first-degree relatives)*	? **(0)** 1 2 PD51
50. **You've said that it doesn't** *[Does it not]* **matter to you what people think of you.** **How do you feel when people praise you or criticize you?**	6. Appears indifferent to the praise or criticism of others. *2 = claims indifference to praise or criticism*	? **(0)** 1 2 PD52
51. **You've said that** *[Do]* **you rarely have strong feelings, like being very angry or feeling joyful.** **Tell me more about that.** *ALSO CONSIDER BEHAVIOR DURING INTERVIEW*	7. Shows emotional coldness, detachment, or flattened affectivity. *2 = not occurring exclusively during a Mood Disorder*	? **(0)** 1 2 PD53

? = Inadequate information   0 = Absent   1 = Subthreshold   2 = Threshold

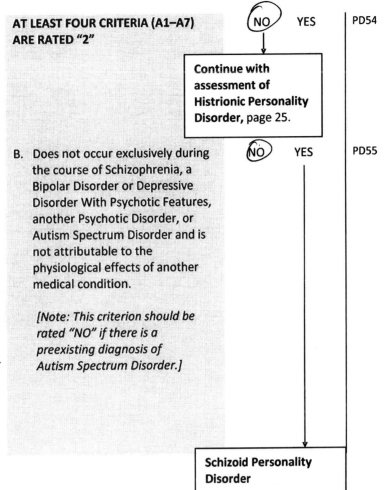

AT LEAST FOUR CRITERIA (A1–A7) ARE RATED "2"   NO   YES   PD54

Continue with assessment of **Histrionic Personality Disorder,** page 25.

IF THERE IS EVIDENCE OF A PSYCHOTIC DISORDER: **Does this happen only when you are having** (SXS OF PSYCHOTIC DISORDER)**?**

IF THERE IS EVIDENCE OF PROLONGED EXCESSIVE ALCOHOL OR DRUG USE THAT RESULTS IN SYMPTOMS THAT RESEMBLE SCHIZOID PD: **Does this happen only when you are drunk or high or withdrawing from alcohol or drugs?**

IF THERE IS EVIDENCE OF A GMC THAT CAUSES SYMPTOMS THAT RESEMBLE SCHIZOID PD: **Were you like that before** (ONSET OF GMC)**?**

B. Does not occur exclusively during the course of Schizophrenia, a Bipolar Disorder or Depressive Disorder With Psychotic Features, another Psychotic Disorder, or Autism Spectrum Disorder and is not attributable to the physiological effects of another medical condition.

[Note: This criterion should be rated "NO" if there is a preexisting diagnosis of Autism Spectrum Disorder.]

NO   YES   PD55

Schizoid Personality Disorder

? = Inadequate information   0 = Absent   1 = Subthreshold   2 = Threshold

HISTRIONIC PERSONALITY DISORDER	HISTRIONIC PERSONALITY DISORDER CRITERIA					

*A pervasive pattern of excessive emotionality and attention seeking, beginning by early adulthood and present in a variety of contexts, as indicated by **five** (or more) of the following:*

52. **You've said that** [Do] **you like being the center of attention.**

How do you feel when you're not? (Uncomfortable?)

1. Is uncomfortable in situations in which he or she is not the center of attention. I'm a performer I need to be on stage.

   2 = feels uncomfortable when not the center of attention

?   0   1   (2)   PD56

53. **You've said that** [Do] **you tend to flirt a lot.**

Has anyone complained about this?

ALSO CONSIDER BEHAVIOR DURING INTERVIEW

2. Interaction with others is often characterized by inappropriate sexually seductive or provocative behavior.

   2 = acknowledges complaints, describes inappropriate behavior, or is observed to be inappropriately seductive

?   0   1   (2)   PD57

54. **You've said that you** [Do you] **often find yourself "coming on" to people.**

Tell me about that.

ALSO CONSIDER BEHAVIOR DURING INTERVIEW

OBSERVED DURING INTERVIEW

From interview observation. Also indicated all his lovers have been upset by this.

3. Displays rapidly shifting and shallow expression of emotions.

?   (0)   1   2   PD58

55. **You've said that you** [Do you] **like to draw attention to yourself by the way you dress or look.**

Describe what you do.

Do you do that kind of thing most of the time?

OBSERVED DURING INTERVIEW

4. Consistently uses physical appearance to draw attention to self.

   2 = gives example and acknowledges that behavior occurs most of the time

It's my style. Also observation.

?   0   1   (2)   PD59

5. Has a style of speech that is excessively impressionistic and lacking in detail. Observed

?   0   1   (2)   PD60

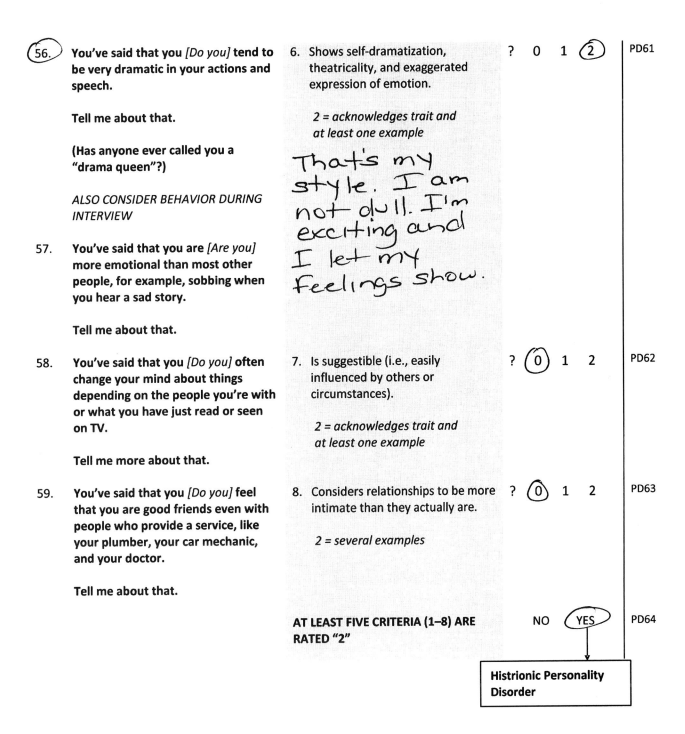

56. **You've said that you [Do you] tend to be very dramatic in your actions and speech.**

    Tell me about that.

    (Has anyone ever called you a "drama queen"?)

    ALSO CONSIDER BEHAVIOR DURING INTERVIEW

57. **You've said that you are [Are you] more emotional than most other people, for example, sobbing when you hear a sad story.**

    Tell me about that.

58. **You've said that you [Do you] often change your mind about things depending on the people you're with or what you have just read or seen on TV.**

    Tell me more about that.

59. **You've said that you [Do you] feel that you are good friends even with people who provide a service, like your plumber, your car mechanic, and your doctor.**

    Tell me about that.

6. Shows self-dramatization, theatricality, and exaggerated expression of emotion.

   2 = acknowledges trait and at least one example

   That's my style. I am not dull. I'm exciting and I let my feelings show.

   ?   0   1   ②   PD61

7. Is suggestible (i.e., easily influenced by others or circumstances).

   2 = acknowledges trait and at least one example

   ?   ⓪   1   2   PD62

8. Considers relationships to be more intimate than they actually are.

   2 = several examples

   ?   ⓪   1   2   PD63

AT LEAST FIVE CRITERIA (1–8) ARE RATED "2"   NO   ⟨YES⟩   PD64

┌─────────────────────────┐
│ **Histrionic Personality** │
│ **Disorder**   │
└─────────────────────────┘

? = Inadequate information   0 = Absent   1 = Subthreshold   2 = Threshold

NARCISSISTIC PERSONALITY DISORDER	NARCISSISTIC PERSONALITY DISORDER CRITERIA					

*A pervasive pattern of grandiosity (in fantasy or behavior), need for admiration, and lack of empathy, beginning by early adulthood and present in a variety of contexts, as indicated by **five** (or more) of the following:*

60. **You've said that you are** *[Are you]* **more important, more talented, or more successful than most other people.**

   Tell me about that.

1. Has a grandiose sense of self-importance (e.g., exaggerates achievements and talents, expects to be recognized as superior without commensurate achievements).

   ? 0 1 ②   PD65

61. **You've said that people have** *[Have people]* **told you that you have too high an opinion of yourself.**

   Give me some examples of this.

   2 = at least one example of grandiosity

   Someday I will have my own fan club.

62. **You've said that** *[Do]* **you think a lot about the power, success, or recognition that you expect to be yours someday.**

   Tell me more about this.

   (How much time do you spend thinking about these things?)

2. Is preoccupied with fantasies of unlimited success, power, brilliance, beauty, or ideal love.

   ? 0 1 ②   PD66

   2 = much of time spent daydreaming or in pursuit of unrealistic goals

   Often daydreams about being a top celebrity.

63. **You've said that** *[Do]* **you think a lot about the perfect romance that will be yours someday.**

   Tell me more about this.

   (How much time do you spend thinking about this?)

64. **You've said that when you have a problem,** *[When you have a problem, do]* **you almost always insist on seeing the top person.** **Give me some examples.** **(Why do you have to see the top person? Is it because you are unique or special? In what way?)**	3. Believes that he or she is "special" and unique and can only be understood by, or should associate with, other special or high-status people (or institutions). *2 = acknowledges that he or she is special or unique and at least one example*	?	0	1	②	PD67

Someone special to understand my problem.

65. **You've said that** *[Do]* **you try to spend time with people who are important or influential.** **Why is that? (Is it because you are too special or unique to spend time with people who are not?)**						

66. **You've said that it is** *[Is it]* **important to you that people pay attention to you or admire you in some way.** **Tell me more about this.**	4. Requires excessive admiration. *2 = acknowledges trait and at least one example*	?	0	1	②	PD68

I need people to recognize my talent

67. **You've said that** *[Do]* **you feel that you are the kind of person who deserves special treatment or that other people should automatically do what you want.** **Tell me about that.**	5. Has a sense of entitlement (i.e., unreasonable expectations of especially favorable treatment or automatic compliance with his or her expectations). *2 = several examples*	?	0	1	②	PD69

wants and deserves free treatment.

68. **You've said that** *[Do]* **you often have to put your needs above other people's.** **Give me some examples of when that happens.**	6. Is interpersonally exploitative (i.e., takes advantage of others to achieve his or her own ends). *2 = several examples in which another person is exploited*	?	0	1	2	PD70

69. **You've said that others have** *[Have others]* **complained that you take advantage of people.** **Tell me about that.**	

? = Inadequate information   0 = Absent   1 = Subthreshold   2 = Threshold

70. **You've said that you** [Do you] **generally feel that other people's needs or feelings are really not your problem.**

    Tell me about that.

71. **You've said that you** [Do you] **often find other people's problems to be boring.**

    Tell me about that.

72. **You've said that people have** [Have people] **complained to you that you don't listen to them or care about their feelings.**

    Tell me about that.

(73.) **You've said that when you see someone who is successful, you** [When you see someone who is successful, do you] **feel that you deserve it more than they do.**

    Give me some examples.
    (How often do you feel that way?)

(74.) **You've said that** [Do] **you feel that others are often envious of you.**

    What do they envy about you?

75. **You've said that you** [Do you] **find that there are very few people who are worth your time and attention.**

    Tell me about that.

    ALSO CONSIDER BEHAVIOR DURING INTERVIEW

76. **You've said that other people have complained** [Have other people complained] **that you act too "high and mighty" or arrogant.**

    Tell me about that.

7. Lacks empathy: is unwilling to recognize or identify with the feelings and needs of others.   ? (0) 1 2   PD71

    2 = acknowledges trait OR several examples

8. Is often envious of others or believes that others are envious of him or her.   ? 0 1 (2)   PD72

    2 = acknowledges trait and at least one example

    I deserve success more than the so called stars. I'm better than they are.

    Most people envy my good looks and style

9. Shows arrogant, haughty behaviors or attitudes.   ? 0 1 (2)   PD73

    2 = acknowledges trait or observed during interview

AT LEAST FIVE CRITERIA (1–9) ARE RATED "2"   NO   (YES)   PD74

Narcissistic Personality Disorder

? = Inadequate information   0 = Absent   1 = Subthreshold   2 = Threshold

BORDERLINE PERSONALITY DISORDER	BORDERLINE PERSONALITY DISORDER CRITERIA					
	*A pervasive pattern of instability of interpersonal relationships, self-image, and affects, and marked impulsivity, beginning by early adulthood and present in a variety of contexts, as indicated by **five** (or more) of the following:*					

77. You've said that you have *[Have you]* become frantic when you thought that someone you really cared about was going to leave you.

What have you done? (Have you threatened or pleaded with him/her?)

How often has this happened?

78. You've said that *[Do]* relationships with people you really care about have lots of extreme ups and downs.

Tell me about them.

(Were there times when you thought these people were perfect or everything you wanted, and then other times when you thought they were terrible? How many relationships have been like this?)

1. Frantic efforts to avoid real or imagined abandonment.

   (**Note:** Do not include suicidal or self-mutilating behavior covered in Criterion 5.)

   2 = several examples
   Happens whenever a relationship is ending. Repeatedly calling ex-lovers.

   ? 0 1 ②   PD75

2. A pattern of unstable and intense interpersonal relationships characterized by alternating between extremes of idealization and devaluation.

   2 = either one prolonged relationship or several briefer relationships in which the alternating pattern occurs at least twice
   Always had stormy relationships

   ? 0 1 ②   PD76

? = Inadequate information   0 = Absent   1 = Subthreshold   2 = Threshold

79. **You've said that your sense of who you are often changes** [*Does your sense of who you are often change*] **dramatically.**

    Tell me more about that.

80. **You've said that you are** [*Are you*] **different with different people or in different situations, so that you sometimes don't know who you really are.**

    Give me some examples of this. (Do you feel this way a lot?)

3. Identity disturbance: markedly and persistently unstable self-image or sense of self.

   [*Note: Do not include normal adolescent uncertainty.*]

   2 = acknowledges trait

   ? (0) 1 2 — PD77

81. **You've said that there have been** [*Have there been*] **lots of sudden changes in your goals, career plans, religious beliefs, and so on.**

    Tell me more about that.

82. **You've said that there have been** [*Have there been*] **lots of sudden changes in the kinds of friends you have or in your sexual identity.**

    Tell me more about that.

(83.) **You've said that you've** [*Have you*] **often done things impulsively.**

    What kinds of things?

    (How about…
    √ …buying things you really couldn't afford?
    √ …having sex with people you hardly knew or having "unsafe sex"?
    √ …drinking too much or taking drugs?
    …driving recklessly?
    …uncontrollable eating?)

    IF YES TO ANY OF ABOVE:
    Tell me about that.
    How often does it happen?

4. Impulsivity in at least two areas that are potentially self-damaging (e.g., spending, sex, substance abuse, reckless driving, binge eating).

   (**Note:** Do not include suicidal or self-mutilating behavior covered in Criterion 5.)

   2 = several examples indicating a pattern of impulsive behavior (not necessarily limited to examples above)

   ? 0 1 (2) — PD78

   Always in credit.
   card debt - drinking
   drugging + sex.

? = Inadequate information   0 = Absent   1 = Subthreshold   2 = Threshold

84. You've said that you have *[Have you]* tried to hurt or kill yourself or threatened to do so.

     IF YES: When was the last time that happened?

5. Recurrent suicidal behavior, gestures, or threats, or self-mutilating behavior.

     2 = two or more events (when not in a Major Depressive Episode)

     [Note: Any current suicidal thoughts, plans, or actions should be thoroughly assessed by the clinician and action taken if necessary.]

?   0   ① 2   PD79

Only once

85. You've said that you have *[Have you ever]* cut, burned, or scratched yourself on purpose.

Tell me about that.

86. You've said that your mood often changes *[Does your mood often change]* in a single day, based on what's going on in your life.

Tell me about that. What kinds of things cause your mood to change?

How long do your "bad" moods typically last?

6. Affective instability due to a marked reactivity of mood (e.g., intense episodic dysphoria, irritability, or anxiety usually lasting a few hours and only rarely more than a few days).

     2 = acknowledges trait

Always extremely moody

?   0   1   ②   PD80

87. You've said that *[Do]* you often feel empty inside.

Tell me more about this.

7. Chronic feelings of emptiness.

     2 = acknowledges trait

?   ⓪   1   2   PD81

88. You've said that *[Do]* you often have temper outbursts or get so angry that you lose control.

Give me some examples.

8. Inappropriate, intense anger or difficulty controlling anger (e.g., frequent displays of temper, constant anger, recurrent physical fights).

     2 = acknowledges trait and at least one example OR several examples

?   ⓪   1   2   PD82

89. You've said that *[Do]* you hit people or throw things when you get angry.

Give me some examples.

(Does this happen often?)

90. You've said that *[Do]* even little things get you very angry.

Give me some examples.

(Does this happen often?)

? = Inadequate information   0 = Absent   1 = Subthreshold   2 = Threshold

91.   **You've said that when you get very upset, you** [When you get very upset, do you] **get suspicious of other people or feel disconnected from your body or that things are unreal.**

In what kinds of situations has this happened?

9. Transient, stress-related paranoid ideation or severe dissociative symptoms.

2 = several stress-related examples that do not occur exclusively during a Psychotic Disorder or a Mood Disorder With Psychotic Features

AT LEAST FIVE CRITERIA (1–9) ARE RATED "2"

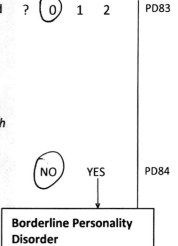

? ⓪ 1 2   PD83

NO   YES   PD84

Borderline Personality Disorder

ANTISOCIAL PERSONALITY DISORDER	ANTISOCIAL PERSONALITY DISORDER CRITERIA					
	B. The individual is at least age 18 years.		NO	(YES)		PD85
[NOTE: FOR A "2" RATING OF ANY CRITERION, THE BEHAVIOR SHOULD NOT OCCUR EXCLUSIVELY DURING THE COURSE OF SCHIZOPHRENIA OR A BIPOLAR DISORDER.]	C. *There is evidence of Conduct Disorder with onset before age 15 years[, as indicated by at least **two** of the following]:*					
92. **You've said that before you were 15, you bullied, threatened, or scared** *[Before you were 15, did you bully, threaten, or scare]* **other kids.** **Give me some examples.** **How often did this happen?**	1. [Before the age of 15] often bullied, threatened, or intimidated others.	?	(0)	1	2	PD86
93. **You've said that before you were 15, you started** *[Before you were 15, did you start]* **fights.** **Give me some examples.** **How often did this happen?**	2. [Before the age of 15] often initiated physical fights.	?	(0)	1	2	PD87
94. **You've said that before you were 15, you hurt or threatened someone** *[Before you were 15, did you hurt or threaten someone]* **with a weapon, like a bat, brick, broken bottle, a knife, or a gun.** **Tell me about that.**	3. [Before the age of 15] has used a weapon that can cause serious physical harm to others (e.g., a bat, brick, broken bottle, knife, gun).	?	(0)	1	2	PD88
95. **You've said that before you were 15, you did** *[Before you were 15, did you do]* **cruel things to someone that caused him or her physical pain or suffering.** **What did you do?**	4. [Before the age of 15] has been physically cruel to people.	?	(0)	1	2	PD89
96. **You've said that before you were 15,** *[Before you were 15, did]* **you hurt animals on purpose.** **What did you do?**	5. [Before the age of 15] has been physically cruel to animals.	?	(0)	1	2	PD90

? = Inadequate information   0 = Absent   1 = Subthreshold   2 = Threshold

97.	You've said that before you were 15, you robbed, mugged, or took *[Before you were 15, did you mug, rob, or forcibly take]* something from someone by threatening him or her. Tell me about that.	6.	[Before the age of 15] has stolen while confronting a victim (e.g., mugging, purse snatching, extortion, armed robbery).	?	(0)	1	2	PD91
98.	You've said that before you were 15, you forced *[Before you were 15, did you force]* someone to do something sexual. Tell me about that.	7.	[Before the age of 15] has forced someone into sexual activity.	?	(0)	1	2	PD92
99.	You've said that before you were 15, *[Before you were 15, did]* you set fires. Tell me about that. Were you hoping to cause serious damage?	8.	[Before the age of 15] has deliberately engaged in fire setting with the intention of causing serious damage.	?	(0)	1	2	PD93
100.	You've said that before you were 15, you deliberately destroyed *[Before you were 15, did you deliberately destroy]* things that weren't yours. What did you do?	9.	[Before the age of 15] has deliberately destroyed others' property (other than by fire setting).	?	(0)	1	2	PD94
101.	You've said that before you were 15, you broke *[Before you were 15, did you break]* into houses, other buildings, or cars. Tell me about that.	10.	[Before the age of 15] has broken into someone else's house, building, or car.	?	(0)	1	2	PD95
102.	You've said that before you were 15, you lied a lot or conned *[Before you were 15, did you lie a lot or con]* other people to get something you wanted or to get out of doing something. Give me some examples. How often did you do that?	11.	[Before the age of 15] often lied to obtain goods or favors or to avoid obligations (i.e., "cons" others).	?	(0)	1	2	PD96

? = Inadequate information   0 = Absent   1 = Subthreshold   2 = Threshold

103. **You've said that before you were 15, you sometimes shoplifted, stole something, or forged** *[Before you were 15, did you sometimes shoplift, steal something, or forge]* **someone's signature for money.**

Give me some examples.

12. [Before the age of 15] has stolen items of nontrivial value without confronting a victim (e.g., shoplifting, [stealing] but without breaking and entering; forgery).

? ⓪ 1 2   PD97

104. **You've said that before you were 15, you ran away from home and stayed** *[Before you were 15, did you run away and stay]* **away overnight.**

Was that more than once?

(With whom were you living at the time?)

13. [Before the age of 15] has run away from home overnight at least twice while living in the parental or parental surrogate home, or once without returning for a lengthy period.

? ⓪ 1 2   PD98

105. **You've said that before you were 13, you would** *[Before you were 13, did you]* **often stay out very late, long after the time you were supposed to be home.**

How often?

14. [Before the age of 13] often stayed out at night despite parental prohibitions.

? ⓪ 1 2   PD99

106. **You've said that before you were 13, you often skipped** *[Before you were 13, did you often skip]* **school.**

How often?

15. [Before the age of 13] was often truant from school.

? ⓪ 1 2   PD100

AT LEAST TWO CONDUCT DISORDER CRITERIA (C1–C15) ARE RATED "2" (i.e., "some symptoms of Conduct Disorder")

NO   YES   PD101

Criterion C of Antisocial Personality Disorder met ("some symptoms of Conduct Disorder"); CONTINUE ON NEXT PAGE.

GO TO *OTHER SPECIFIED PERSONALITY DISORDER,* Page 40.

? = Inadequate information   0 = Absent   1 = Subthreshold   2 = Threshold

[NOTE: FOR A "2" RATING OF ANY CRITERION, THE BEHAVIOR SHOULD NOT OCCUR EXCLUSIVELY DURING THE COURSE OF SCHIZOPHRENIA OR A BIPOLAR DISORDER.]

Now, since you were 15...

Have you done things that are against the law—even if you weren't caught—like stealing, identity theft, writing bad checks, or having sex for money?

IF NOT KNOWN FROM OVERVIEW: **Have you ever been arrested for anything?**

Do you often lie to get what you want or just for the fun of it?

Have you ever used an alias or pretended you were someone else?

Have you "conned" others to get something?

Do you often do something on the spur of the moment without thinking about how it will affect you or other people?

Tell me about that. What kinds of things?

Did you ever walk off a job without having another one to go to? (How many times?)

Have you ever moved out of a place without having another place to live? Tell me about that.

Have you been in any fights? (How often?)

Have you ever been so angry that you hit or threw things at other people (INCLUDING SPOUSE/PARTNER)? (How many times?)

Have you ever hit a child very hard? Tell me about that.

Have you physically threatened or hurt anyone else? Tell me about that. (How often?)

A. *A pervasive pattern of disregard for and violation of the rights of others, occurring since age 15 years, as indicated by* **three** *(or more) of the following:*

	?	0	1	2	
1. Failure to conform to social norms with respect to lawful behaviors, as indicated by repeatedly performing acts that are grounds for arrest. *2 = several examples*	?	(0)	1	2	PD102
2. Deceitfulness, as indicated by repeated lying, use of aliases, or conning others for personal profit or pleasure. *2 = several examples*	?	(0)	1	2	PD103
3. Impulsivity or failure to plan ahead. *2 = several examples*	?	(0)	1	2	PD104
4. Irritability and aggressiveness, as indicated by repeated physical fights or assaults. *2 = several examples*	?	(0)	1	2	PD105

? = Inadequate information   0 = Absent   1 = Subthreshold   2 = Threshold

Did you ever drive a car when you were drunk or high? How many speeding tickets have you gotten or car accidents have you been in? Do you always use protection if you have sex with someone you don't know well? (Has anyone ever said that you allowed a child to be in danger when you were supposed to be taking care of the child?)	5. Reckless disregard for safety of self or others. *2 = several examples*	? ⓪ 1 2	PD106
How much of the time in the last 5 years were you not working? *IF FOR A PROLONGED PERIOD*: **Why?** (Was there work available?) When you were working, did you miss a lot of work? *IF YES:* **Why?** Have you ever owed people money and not paid them back? (How often?) What about not paying child support or not giving money to children or someone else who depended on you?	6. Consistent irresponsibility, as indicated by repeated failure to sustain consistent work behavior or honor financial obligations. *2 = several examples*	? ⓪ 1 2	PD107
IF THERE IS EVIDENCE OF ANTISOCIAL ACTS AND IT IS UNCLEAR WHETHER THERE IS ANY REMORSE: **How do you feel about** (ANTISOCIAL ACTS)? (Do you think what you did was wrong in any way?) Do you think you were justified in (ANTISOCIAL ACTS)? (Do you think the other person deserved it?)	7. Lack of remorse, as indicated by being indifferent to or rationalizing having hurt, mistreated, or stolen from another. *2 = lacks remorse about several antisocial acts*	? ⓪ 1 2	PD108

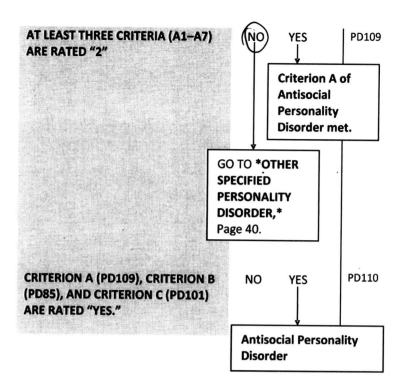

OTHER SPECIFIED PERSONALITY DISORDER

OTHER SPECIFIED PERSONALITY DISORDER CRITERIA

[A presentation] in which symptoms characteristic of a personality disorder... predominate but do not meet the full criteria for any of the disorders in the Personality Disorders diagnostic class.

NO   YES   PD111

END OF SCID-5-PD. FILL OUT DIAGNOSTIC SUMMARY SCORE SHEET ON PAGE 1.

What problems has this caused for you?

Has this affected your relationships or your interactions with other people?

How about your family, romantic partner or friends?

Has this affected you work/school?

Has it bothered other people?

[The presentation causes] clinically significant distress or impairment in social, occupational, or other important areas of functioning.

NO   YES

Other Specified Personality Disorder

END OF SCID-5-PD. FILL OUT DIAGNOSTIC SUMMARY SCORE SHEET ON PAGE 1.